CORE TOPICS IN AIRWAY MANAGEMENT

This book provides an easy-to-read introduction to this important topic that will be of value to a wide spectrum of healthcare professionals including anaesthetists, intensivists, Operating Department Practitioners (ODPs), theatre and recovery nurses. Concise but comprehensive chapters from experts in the field cover everything from basic anatomy, physiology and applied physics through to the various methods of maintaining the airway under anaesthesia such as the facemask, supraglottic devices and tracheal intubation by various methods with single or double-lumen tubes. The problem airway is also discussed in detail including obstruction by infection, tumour or a foreign body, the shared airway in ENT and maxillofacial surgery, aspiration, problems in obstetrics, trauma, cervical spine disease, intensive care, the 'lost' airway, paediatrics, extubation and recovery. Additional valuable chapters cover the specification and design of standard and laser-proof tracheal tubes, decontamination of airway equipment, the nature and treatment of morbidity and important medico-legal issues.

To Dr Archie Brain

CORE TOPICS IN AIRWAY MANAGEMENT

Edited by

Ian Calder
Consultant Anaesthetist
The National Hospital for Neurology and The Royal Free Hospital
London

Adrian Pearce
Consultant Anaesthetist
Guy's and St Thomas' Hospital
London

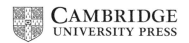
CAMBRIDGE
UNIVERSITY PRESS

CAMBRIDGE UNIVERSITY PRESS
Cambridge, New York, Melbourne, Madrid, Cape Town, Singapore, São Paulo

Cambridge University Press
The Edinburgh Building, Cambridge CB2 8RU, UK

Published in the United States of America by Cambridge University Press, New York

www.cambridge.org
Information on this title: www.cambridge.org/9780521869102

First published 2005
Reprinted with corrections 2006
Reprinted 2007

Printed in the United Kingdom at the University Press, Cambridge

A catalog record for this publication is available from the British Library

ISBN-13 978-0-521-86910-2 hardback

Every effort has been made in preparing this book to provide accurate and
up-to-date information that is in accord with accepted standards and
practice at the time of publication. Nevertheless, the authors, editors and
publisher can make no warranties that the information contained herein is
totally free from error, not least because clinical standards are constantly
changing through research and regulation. The authors, editors and
publisher therefore disclaim all liability for direct or consequential
damages resulting from the use of material contained in this book. Readers
are strongly advised to pay careful attention to information provided by the
manufacturer of any drugs or equipment that they plan to use.

CONTENTS

LIST OF CONTRIBUTORS

Pieter A.J. Borg
Consultant Anaesthetist
University Hospital of Maastricht
Netherlands

Ian Calder
Consultant Anaesthetist
The National Hospital for Neurology and The Royal
Free Hospital
London

Tim Cook
Consultant Anaesthetist
The Royal United Hospital
Bath

Bert Dercksen
Consultant Anaesthetist
Wilhemina Ziekenhuis
Assen
Netherlands

Adrian Pearce
Consultant Anaesthetist
Guy's and St Thomas' Hospital
London

John Picard
Consultant Anaesthetist
Charing Cross Hospital
London

Andrew D. Farmery
Consultant Anaesthetist
The John Radcliffe Hospital
Oxford

Peter Ford
Specialist Registrar in Anaesthesia
The Gloucestershire Royal NHS Trust
Gloucester

Chris Frerk
Consultant Anaesthetist
Northampton General Hospital
Northampton

David A. Gabbott
Consultant Anaesthetist
The Gloucestershire Royal NHS Trust
Gloucester

Hamish Gray
Consultant Anaesthetist
Christchurch
New Zealand

John Henderson
Consultant Anaesthetist
The Western Infirmary
Glasgow

Viki Mitchell
Consultant Anaesthetist
The Middlesex Hospital
London

Anil Patel
Consultant Anaesthetist
The Royal National ENT Hospital
London

Om Sanehi
Consultant Anaesthetist
Trafford and Salford Hospital
Manchester

Adrian Steele
Consultant Anaesthetist
Charing Cross Hospital
London

Peter J.H. Venn
Consultant Anaesthetist
The Queen Victoria Hospital
East Grinstead

Richard Vanner
Consultant Anaesthetist
The Gloucestershire Royal NHS Trust
Gloucester

Steve M. Yentis
Consultant Anaesthetist
The Chelsea and Westminster Hospital
London

Rob W.M. Walker
Consultant Anaesthetist
Booth Hall Children's Hospital
Manchester

PREFACE

Every anaesthetist will reach the end of his/her career with a collection of difficult airway experiences. There can be few more terrifying experiences in medical practice than the realization that a cyanosed patient is getting worse, not better, particularly when the patient was nice and pink before the anaesthetic began. Many seasoned anaesthetists recognize the change that comes over trainees after their first experience of serious difficulty with the airway. One of the editors remembers a conversation with a distinguished American paediatric anaesthetist about the difficulty of keeping up with bright young residents. Her observation that *'a few deep paediatric desaturations sure does take the shine off 'em'* was correct. All of us who have been around for some time have 'been there', and we know we could find ourselves in difficulty any time we give an anaesthetic.

Management of the airway of patients who are sedated, obtunded or anaesthetized is the responsibility of nursing and medical practitioners in anaesthesia, emergency medicine, intensive care medicine and other critical care areas. Anaesthetists do not own the airway and their right to be considered expert can be based only on good clinical practice, knowledge of relevant basic science and critical evaluation of every component of airway care.

There is an uneasy combination of science and art in airway management. We know a good deal about the physics and physiology, but are less certain about the safest way to manage the airway in many patients. Meetings of the *Difficult Airway Society* have often been lacking in consensus, sometimes confusing, but always educational. It is probably just that there really are several ways to pluck a chicken. However, there are core topics, which anyone who professes to be an anaesthetist should be aware of, and our purpose in writing this book is to present this material. We hope that there is little excess fat in this book and that it represents core knowledge that readers of all levels of experience will find valuable.

Ian Calder
Adrian Pearce
July 2004

ACKNOWLEDGEMENTS

The editors would like to thank the Audio-visual Departments of the National Hospital and the Royal Free Hospital, and Samantha Churchill and Rob Bailey of Keymed Ltd.

LIST OF ABBREVIATIONS

AAGBA	Association of Anaesthetists of Great Britain and Ireland
ADP	Adenosine Diphosphate
AMBU	Airway Mask Breathing Unit
AMD™	Airway Management Device
AP	Anterio-Posterior
APL	Adjustable Pressure Limiting
ARDS	Acute Respiratory Distress Syndrome
ASA	American Society of Anesthesiologists
ATP	Adenosine Triphosphate
BIPAP	Bilevel Positive Airway Pressure
BMI	Body Mass Index
BMJ	British Medical Journal
BP	Blood Pressure
BS	British Standards
BURP	Pressure Applied Backwards, Upwards and to the Right
CCTV	Closed Circuit Television
CICO	Can't Intubate Can't Oxygenate
CJD	Creutzfeldt-Jakob Disease
cLMA	Classic Laryngeal Mask Airway
CobraPLA™	Cobra Perilaryngeal Airway
COSHH	Control of Substances Hazardous to Health
CPAP	Continuous Positive Airway Pressure
CPB	Cardiopulmonary Bypass
CSF	Cerebrospinal Fluid
CT	Computerized Tomography
CTM	Cricothyroid Membrane
CVCI	Can't Ventilate Can't Intubate
CVS	Cardiovascular System
DAS	Difficult Airway Society
DLTs	Double Lumen Tubes
ECG	Electrocardiogram
EDS	Excessive Day-Time Sleepiness
EEG	Electroencephalogram
ELM	External Laryngeal Manipulation
EMG	Electromyographic

EN	European Standards
ENT	Ear, Nose and Throat
EPP	Equal Pressure Point
ET/ETT	Endotracheal Tube
ETVC	Endotracheal Ventilation Catheter
EU	European Union
FDA	Food and Drug Administration
FRC	Functional Residual Capacity
FV	Flow Volume
GCS	Glasgow Coma Scale
GI	Gastrointestinal
GTN	Glyceryl Trinitrate
Hb	Haemoglobin
HDU	High Dependency Unit
HP	Hypopharynx
HPV	Hypoxic Pulmonary Vasoconstriction
HR	Heart Rate
ICP	Intracranial Pressure
ICU	Intensive Care Unit
ID	Internal/Inner Diameter
ILCOR	International Liaison Committee on Resuscitation
ILMA™	Intubating Laryngeal Mask Airway
IPPV	Intermittent Positive Pressure Ventilation
ISO	International Organization for Standardization
IT	Implant Testing
ITU	Intensive Therapy Unit
I.V.	Intravenous
L	Larynx
LMA	Laryngeal Mask Airway
LOS	Line of Sight
LR	Likelihood Ratio
LT®	Laryngeal Tube
LTS®	Laryngeal Tube Sonda
MILS	Manual In-Line Stabilization
MRI	Magnetic Resonance Imaging
NADH	Nicotinamide Adenine Dinucleotide
nCPAP	Nasal Continuous Positive Airway Pressure
NIBP	Non-Invasive Blood Pressure
NIV	Non-Invasive Ventilation
NP	Nasopharynx

OGT	Orogastric Tube
OP	Oropharynx
OSA	Obstructive Sleep Apnoea
PACU	Post-Anaesthesia Care Unit
PAx™	Pharyngeal Airway xpress
P_c	Pressure at Site of Collapsible Segment
PCT	Percutaneous Tracheostomy
PCV	Pollution Control Valve
P_d	Downstream Pressure
PEEP	Positive End Expiratory Pressure
PICU	Paediatric Intensive Care Unit
PLMA™	ProSeal Laryngeal Mask Airway
POGO	Percentage of Glottic Opening
PPV	Positive Predictive Value
PSG	Polysomnogram
P_t	Tissue Pressure
P_u	Upstream Pressure
PVC	Polyvinyl Chloride
RAE	Ring-Adair-Elwyn
REM	Rapid Eye Movement
RSI	Rapid Sequence Induction
RTA	Road Traffic Accident
SADs	Supraglottic Airway Devices
SCI	Spinal Cord Injury
SCIWORA	Spinal Cord Injury Without Radiographic Abnormality
SLIPA	Streamlined Liner of the Pharynx Airway
SP	Soft Palate
TCI	Target-Controlled Infusion
TLC	Total Lung Capacity
TMJ	Temporo-Mandibular Joint
TNG	Tongue
TNM	Tumour, Necrosis and Metastasis
TTJV	Transtracheal Jet Ventilation
UPPP	Uvulopalatopharyngoplasty
vCJD	Variant Creutzfeldt-Jakob Disease
VIPs	Very Important Persons
VP	Velopharynx
V/Q	Ventilation/Perfusion

ANATOMY

1

J. Picard

Fine lingerie itself is rather tedious: it is the context that makes it exciting. The same is true for anatomy: topology alone is for idiots-savants. The following lines instead offer a selective account of the functional anatomy of the adult head, neck and airway as it applies to anaesthetic clinical practice.

The mouth

The mouth is dominated by the tongue, a muscular instrument of pleasure – gastronomic and linguistic. For anaesthetists, little else counts but its size. It may be swollen acutely (as in angioneurotic oedema), but is also susceptible to disproportionate enlargement in trisomy 21, myxoedema, acromegaly and glycogen storage diseases, among others.

Angioneurotic oedema can cause such swelling as to fill the entire pharynx, preventing both nasal and mouth breathing and making a percutaneous subglottic airway necessary for survival. Less dramatically, a large tongue (relative to the submandibular space) can hinder direct laryngoscopy. That is, manoeuvered with reasonable force, the laryngoscope blade should squeeze the posterior tongue so as to allow a direct view of the glottis. If the tongue is too large, or the jaw hypotrophied, it may not be possible to see the glottis over the compressed tongue.

Within the mouth, the tongue is like a thrust stage in a theatre. It is surrounded by two tiers of teeth (stalls and royal circle), and a series of trapdoors, wings and flies (Figure 1.1).

Each tooth consists of calcified dentine, cementum and enamel surrounding a cavity filled (if the tooth is alive) with vessels and nerves. Each tooth is held in its socket in the jaw by a periodontal ligament. If a tooth is inadvertently knocked out, the sooner it is returned to its socket the better. If the root is clean, the tooth can simply be put back in; if dirty, the root should first be rinsed with saline or whole milk. A dentist will then be able to splint the tooth in place. If a displaced tooth cannot be immediately replaced, whole milk is the best storage medium; a dental cavity exposed too long to saline, or worse water, dies. Calcification of the periodontal ligament is then inevitable, and the tooth will become brittle and discoloured, and may fracture, loosen or fall out again.

The floor of the mouth can be opened like a trap by a surgeon. During maxillo-facial surgery, for example, oral and nasal tubes may both obstruct surgical access. (Fractures may further relatively contraindicate nasal intubation.) If long-term ventilatory support is unlikely, then a tracheostomy can be avoided by a submandibular intubation: a plane is developed from the submandibular triangle (between anterior and posterior bellies of digastric) to the floor of the mouth, avoiding the salivary apparatus and the lingual nerve, and a tracheal tube passed from the oral cavity despite the closed mouth.

The stage's side wings are formed by mucosal folds running over palatoglossal and palatopharyngeal muscles (from anterior backwards). Between the two folds on each side lie the tonsils (which may be invisible in adults, but in children may be so large as to kiss in the midline, hampering laryngoscopy). The glossopharyngeal nerve runs under the mucosa of the base of the palatoglossal arch (towards the posterior tongue) and can be blocked there. (Just as in the theatre, so in the mouth: confusion

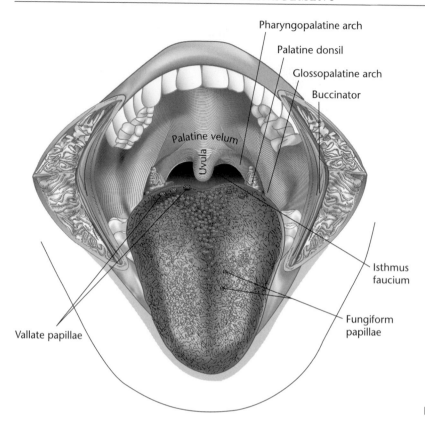

Figure 1.1 The mouth.

surrounds the wings. Properly called the palatoglossal and palatopharyngeal arches, they are also commonly called *fauces and pillars*. They are all the same thing.)

Access to the stage's flies is controlled by the soft palate, a flap of soft tissue which can move up to separate the nasopharynx from the mouth and oropharynx (during swallowing), or move down to separate/shield the pharynx from mouth (during chewing).

The nose

The nose has evolved to humidify and warm air before directing it to the nasopharynx and thence towards the lungs; all roles likely to be subverted by anaesthetists. Nevertheless the anatomy of both inside and outside of the nose has anaesthetic relevance.

The nose encases the two nasal cavities which each lead from nostril to nasopharynx. Each cavity is lined by a mucous membrane of peculiar vascularity; this luxurient perfusion limits local cooling and dessication despite evaporation. It also means minimal trauma can cause profuse bleeding.

The mucosa's innervation is so complex as to make topical anaesthesia the most practical option for even the most ardent regional anaesthetist (no less than nine nerves innervate each cavity). That said, simply pouring a local anaesthetic solution down the nostrils of a supine anaesthetized patient is profoundly unanatomical: the solution can be directed to its target by gravity. Before functional endoscopic sinus surgery, for example, if the solution is to reach the cephalad, reaches of the nasal cavity, the head must be tilted back (with Trendelenburg tilt and a pillow below the shoulders). To direct solution along the projected path of a fibrescope, less Trendelenburg is necessary. Moreover, some

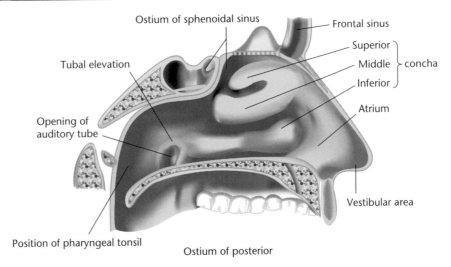

Figure 1.2 The lateral nose.

sensory fibres pass through the contralateral spheno-palatine ganglion. It is therefore sensible to apply local anaesthetic to both nostrils, even if only one is to be subjected to a foreign body.

Each nasal cavity is divided by three turbinates (more properly conchae) which extend laterally from the midline (Figure 1.2). The space between the floor of the nose and the inferior concha is larger than that between inferior and middle conchae. Moreover the more caudad a fibrescope's path, the less acutely it must turn past the soft palate towards the glottis. For both reasons, keeping a 'scope to the floor' of the nose should facilitate its passage. Furthermore, the ostia (holes) through which the sinuses drain into the nose are all cepha-lad to the inferior concha. A foreign body running caudad to it may therefore be less likely to obstruct drainage or cause sinusitis.

The damage that can be done by tubes passed blindly through the nose is remarkable; entire conchae have been amputated, and the brain directly oxygenated by tubes passed into it through fractures in the skull base. Clearly endotracheal tubes should be of as small a diameter as possible while bleeding diatheses and basal skull fractures are contraindications to nasal intubation. The nose's profile also determines how tightly a face mask can

fit. Too large a nasal bone, gas escapes around the mask's sides, and too small, gas escapes at the midline.

Glottis and epiglottis

The human larynx is often declared the organ of speech (Figure 1.3). More extraordinary, still it allows singing. Its intrinsic musculature is accord-ingly complex, but not always relevant to the anaes-thetist simply aiming for the cavity the muscles surround. That said, a naming of the parts seen on laryngoscopy allows accurate description of abnor-mality. Just as for a glutton before fancy chocolates, only a few details of the box are relevant; the key is to get in, past the epiglottis and past the cords themselves.

The epiglottis has evolved to shield the glottis not from anaesthetists, but from nutrients headed towards the stomach. It works like the flexible lid of a pedal bin. Generally it is half open, to allow respir-ation. But on swallowing the epiglottis and larynx come together. Like the lid closing on the bin, the larger and more flexible the epiglottis, the better it can fit the glottis, but the more it can frustrate direct laryngoscopy. Given adequate anaesthesia, the

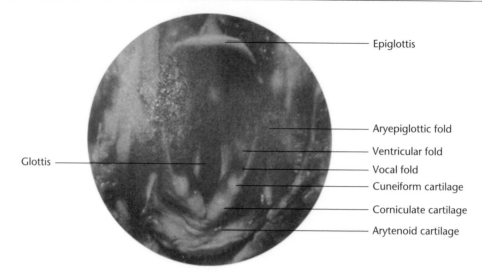

Figure 1.3 Anatomic specimen of adult human larynx.

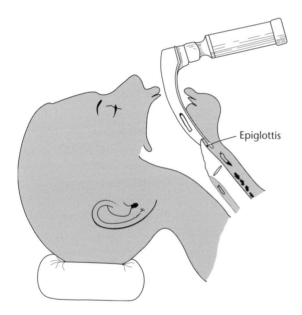

Figure 1.4 The laryngoscope.

tip of a laryngoscope placed in the vallecula and drawn anteriorly will generally also pull the epiglottis sufficiently far anteriorly to reveal the glottis. But if an anaesthetized patient is in the supine position, and the epiglottis is long and flaccid, it may fall to hide the cords unless it too is scooped above the laryngoscope's blade (Figure 1.4).

The mucosa of the larynx above the cords is supplied by the internal laryngeal nerve; below the cords, the mucosa is innervated by the recurrent laryngeal nerve, which also supplies all the intrinsic muscles of the larynx (bar cricothyroid, innervated by the external laryngeal nerve). As it is purely sensory, the internal laryngeal nerve can be blocked without fear of attendant paresis. But transection of the recurrent laryngeal nerve partially adducts the cord, and – worse – less extreme surgical damage of the nerve can cause the cord to adduct more extremely, across the midline. So anatomy dictates that the mucosa below the cords is anaesthetized topically, if at all.

Subglottic airway: cricothyroid puncture and tracheostomy

'If you cannot go through it, go round it': if teeth, tongue, epiglottis or glottis obstruct the path to the cords, then it may be easier to reach the trachea directly through skin, either by cricothyroid puncture or tracheostomy.

As the trachea must run posteriorly from the glottis to reach the carina in the mediastinum, it is most superficial at its start. Indeed, the defect between the thyroid cartilage and the first tracheal ring (the cricoid) is easily palpable in a normal neck, and is covered only by skin, loose areolar

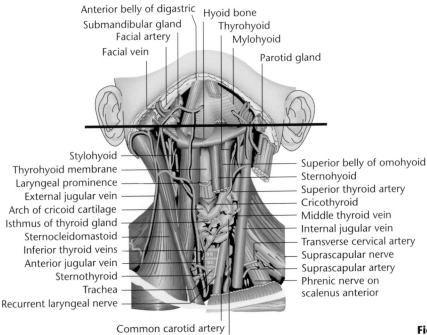

Anterior belly of digastric
Submandibular gland
Facial artery
Facial vein
Hyoid bone
Thyrohyoid
Mylohyoid
Parotid gland

Stylohyoid
Thyrohyoid membrane
Laryngeal prominence
External jugular vein
Arch of cricoid cartilage
Isthmus of thyroid gland
Sternocleidomastoid
Inferior thyroid veins
Anterior jugular vein
Sternothyroid
Trachea
Recurrent laryngeal nerve

Superior belly of omohyoid
Sternohyoid
Superior thyroid artery
Cricothyroid
Middle thyroid vein
Internal jugular vein
Transverse cervical artery
Suprascapular nerve
Suprascapular artery
Phrenic nerve on
scalenus anterior

Common carotid artery
Lateral lobe of thyroid gland

Figure 1.5 Thyroid gland and the front of the neck.

tissue and the fibrous cricothyroid membrane (Figure 1.5). So, in theory, a needle or cannula can be passed into the trachea here without risk of haemorrhage from anterior structures. But posteriorly the oesophagus runs directly behind the trachea, and the needle can perforate the posterior wall of the trachea. Moreover, the gap between cricoid and thyroid cartilages will not admit a tube wide enough to allow conventional ventilation: some form of jetting device must be used.

More caudally a larger tube can be passed into the trachea without undue force (either surgically or with a percutaneous technique). But again the oesophagus runs directly behind the trachea, and can be damaged through the posterior wall in a percutaneous approach. Moreover, the trachea is far from subcutaneous as it approaches the sternum: the thyroid isthmus lies over the second, third and fourth tracheal rings; from there the inferior thyroid veins drain the gland running close to the midline towards the chest – and in a short neck, the left brachiocephalic vein may poke above the sternum as it crosses the trachea.

Trachea and bronchial tree

Like a jetliner's wing, the trachea's apparent simplicity belies its complexity. It is held open by the tracheal cartilages. The most cephalad of these (the cricoid) forms a complete ring. (Indeed, cricoid means 'like a ring'.) The remainder are each shaped like a C, with the curve facing anteriorly. Not only does this help disorientated bronchoscopists, it also allows the tracheal bore to vary. The two ends of each C are joined by the trachealis muscle which forms the posterior wall of the trachea. If the muscle tightens the trachea's radius is reduced (as the points of the C are drawn together), airway resistance rises and the volume of the dead space falls; conversely, airway resistance falls and the dead space swells as the muscle relaxes. So, just as in a wing, the trachea's shape can be optimized for different flow rates (Figure 1.6).

As the bronchial tree ramifies beyond the trachea, its initial divisions are crucially asymmetric. The carina itself is on the left of the midline; the left main bronchus is narrower and runs off closer to

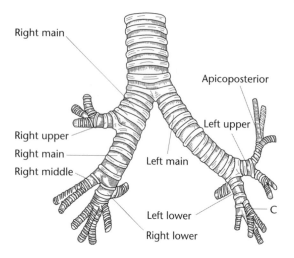

Figure 1.6 Main, lobar and segmental bronchi.

the horizontal than the right; all conspire to send aspirated material towards the right main bronchus. Moreover, in an adult the left main bronchus is some 4.5 cm long while the right main bronchus runs just 2.5 cm before giving off the bronchus to the right upper lobe. Clearly a larger target is easier to hit. It is therefore easier to isolate the lungs without occluding a lobar bronchus, if the left rather than the right main bronchus is the target.

Mouth opening and the temporo-mandibular joint

Hominids evolved before cutlery: so, until the Stone Age, biting hard and opening the mouth wide were both advantageous.

A strong bite and a wide gape may seem to be conflicting ambitions. A firm bite, for instance, depends on a single-fused mandible, and on muscles inserting some way from the joint to gain greater leverage, as in humans (Figure 1.7). (In snakes, in contrast, each of the two halves of the mandible and the maxilla move independently from the skull and from each other, and their muscles insert close to the relevant joints, to give an enormous gape, but weak bite.)

An adequate gape is nevertheless achieved in most humans by subluxation. When the jaw is closed, the

(a)

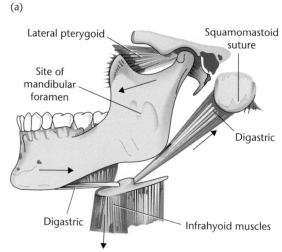

(b)

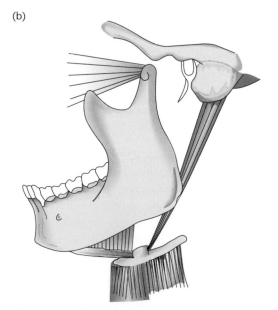

Figure 1.7 (a) Mandible and muscle actions. (b) Mandibular movement for opening the mouth wide.

head of the mandible rests in the mandibular fossa in the temporal bone. But as the jaw opens, the head of the mandible is pulled out of the fossa by the lateral pterygoids. Rather than turning on its head, the mandible swivels on an axis which runs through the mandibular foramina (i.e. close to the insertion sites of temporalis and masseter). This shift in the axis of rotation allows both strong bite and wide gape: at the limit of closure, as the molars meet, the jaw is turning on the temporo-mandibular joint, and masseter and temporalis are working with leverage. But at the jaw's widest opening, it turns about their insertion sites; they are not so passively stretched and the bones of the joint do not so impinge on one another. The lower limit of normal inter-incisor distance has been found to be 37 mm in young adults. Mouth opening declines with age and in general females have slightly smaller inter-incisor distances.

Mouth opening ability also depends on cranio-cervical flexion/extension. Head extension facilitates opening. Normal humans extend about 26° from the neutral position at the cranio-cervical junction to achieve maximal mouth opening. If extension from the neutral position is prevented a subject can be expected to lose about one third of their normal inter-dental distance. Patients with poor cranio-cervical extension therefore suffer a 'double whammy' in terms of airway management.

Cervical spine

Mobility and strength also characterize the cervical spine. The mobility stems from the arrangement of so many bones over a comparatively short distance (as at the wrist); the strength from the geometry of the joints' articular surfaces and from the ligaments which bind them.

The joints between occiput, atlas (C1) and axis (C2) are unlike others in the vertebral column. Working caudad, the occipital condyles rest on the lateral masses of atlas like the rails of a rocking horse stuck in tram tracks: the head can flex forward at the joint (until the odontoid hits the skull) and extend backwards; some abduction is allowed, but rotation is not possible. Atlas, however, turns around the axial odontoid peg. Posterior movement of atlas over axis is obviously limited by the axial anterior arch impinging on the peg (Figure 1.8).

Otherwise ligaments are responsible for the stability of the joints:

- the alar ligaments run from the sides of the peg to the foramen magnum – depending on which

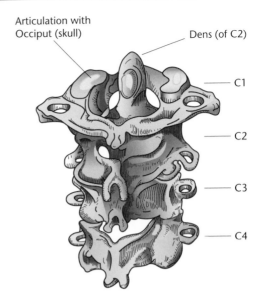

Figure 1.8 Atlas and axis.

Articulation with Occiput (skull)

Dens (of C2)

C1

C2

C3

C4

way the head is turned, one or other tightens and so limits rotation;
- the transerve band of the cruciform ligament runs behind the peg, from one side of atlas to the other – it stops atlas moving anteriorly over axis;
- the tectorial membrane runs as a fibrous sheet from the back of the body of the peg to insert around the anterior half of the foramen magnum – running anterior to the axis around which the head nods, it tightens as the head is extended.

The functional unit formed by the base of the skull, the atlas and the axis, is often known as the 'occipito-atlanto-axial complex'. Normal movement at this complex permits easy airway management, both for mask anaesthesia ('chin lift') and direct laryngoscopy. Quantification of the movements of the cervical spine is not simple. There is considerable variation in the population and the range of all movements declines with age. Wilson suggested the use of a pencil placed on, and at right angles to, the forehead. The angle swept by the pencil during flexion/extension should be more than 80°. Another method is to compare the movement of a line between the canthus of the eye and tragus of the ear and also a horizontal or vertical line. The normal range of extension from the neutral position is about 60°. An attractive but sadly, generally impractical, test is to ask the subject to drink from a narrow champagne flute. Patients with poor cranio-cervical movement find this difficult.

Below the axis, in the 'subaxial' spine, the vertebrae assume a more conventional form. They articulate at the zygapophyseal joints between each bone's facets. Extension and flexion are both limited by the bones impinging on one another, either at the facet joints, or in the anterior midline.

Like the other subjects in this chapter, the normal cervical spine is largely relevant only to the extent that it obstructs anaesthetists' access to the airway. Direct laryngoscopy is classically facilitated by bringing oral, pharyngeal and laryngeal axes into line. In practice that means extension at the occipito-atlanto-axial complex and minimal movement in the subaxial cervical spine.

Key points

- The landmarks associated with the cricothyroid membrane offer the easiest emergency site for percutaneous airway access.
- The oesophagus lies behind the trachea and is easily perforated by needles introduced into the trachea.

- Normal mouth opening is a complex phenomenon.
- The occipito-atlanto-axial complex has a profound influence on airway management.

Further reading

Calder I, Picard J, Chapman M, O'Sullevan C, Crockard HA. Mouth opening – a new angle. *Anesthesiology* 2003; **99**: 799–801.

Crosby ET. Airway management after upper cervical spine injury: what have we learned? *Can J Anaesth* 2002; **49**: 733–744.

Hernández AF. The submental route for endotracheal intubation. A new technique. *J Max Fac Surg* 1986; **14**: 64–65.

Pemberton P, Calder I, O'Sullivan C, Crockard HA. The champagne angle. *Anaesthesia* 2002; **57**: 402–403.

Sawin PD, Todd MM, Traynelis VC *et al.* Cervical spine motion with direct laryngoscopy and orotracheal intubation: an *in vivo* cinefluoroscopic study of subjects without cervical abnormality. *Anesthesiology* 1996; **85**: 26–36.

Sinnatamby CS. *Last's Anatomy: Regional and Applied.* Edinburgh: *Churchill Livingstone*, 1999.

PHYSIOLOGY OF APNOEA AND HYPOXIA 2

A.D. Farmery

Ethical constraints make the study of this all important topics very difficult. Simple questions, such as *how long will an apnoeic patient survive?* – cannot be answered with precision.

Classification of hypoxia

'Cellular respiration' occurs at the level of the mitochondria, when electrons are passed from an electron donor (reduced nicotinamide adenine dinucleotide (NADH)) via the mitochondrial respiratory cytochromes to 'reduce' molecular oxygen (O_2). The energy from this redox reaction is used to phosphorylate adenosine diphosphate (ADP), thereby generating the universal energy source, adenosine triphosphate (ATP), which powers all biological processes. If molecular O_2 cannot be reduced in this way, this bit of biochemistry fails and cellular hypoxia occurs. Based on Barcroft's original classification, four separate causes of cellular hypoxia can be considered. Three of these four factors affect O_2 delivery to the tissues ($\dot{D}O_2$), which is described mathematically by the equation in Box 2.1. Derangements of each of the terms on the right-hand side of this equation will reduce O_2 delivery to tissues.

The fourth cause of cellular hypoxia in our classification is *histotoxic hypoxia*. An example of this is cyanide or carbon monoxide poisoning. In histotoxic hypoxia, there is not (or there need not be) any deficit in O_2 delivery. Cellular and mitochondrial partial pressure of O_2 (PO_2) may be more than adequate, but the deficit lies in the reduction of molecular O_2 due to a failure of electron transfer. In order to fully understand the classification of hypoxia, it is useful to consider the example of carbon monoxide poisoning.

What is the mechanism of death in severe carbon monoxide poisoning?

After an unsuccessful suicide attempt involving motor exhaust-gas inhalation, a patient is taken to hospital. He is alert and breathing O_2 enriched air via a Hudson mask. His haemoglobin concentration is $15\,g\,dl^{-1}$, and his carboxyhaemoglobin fraction is 33%. The patient later dies. What is the mechanism of his death?

Let us consider each of the factors of Barcroft's classification in Box 2.1.

Hypoxaemic hypoxia is not likely to be the cause. Assuming no lung damage has occurred, this patient's arterial (P_aO_2) is likely to be normal if breathing air, or elevated if breathing O_2. P_aO_2 is determined by the gas-exchanging properties of the lung, and is unaffected by haemoglobin concentration or by the nature of the haemoglobin species present.

A common (and erroneous) answer to this question is that, since carbon monoxide has a very high affinity for haemoglobin, and that since carboxyhaemoglobin has no O_2 carrying capacity, O_2 delivery to tissues is compromised, resulting in cellular hypoxia and death. This is clearly erroneous since if total haemoglobin concentration is $15\,g\,dl^{-1}$ and the carboxyhaemoglobin fraction is 33% then there is $10\,g\,dl^{-1}$ of normal haemoglobin which, since the P_aO_2 is normal, is fully saturated. While this does constitute a form of functional anaemia, an *anaemic hypoxia* mechanism cannot realistically be implicated

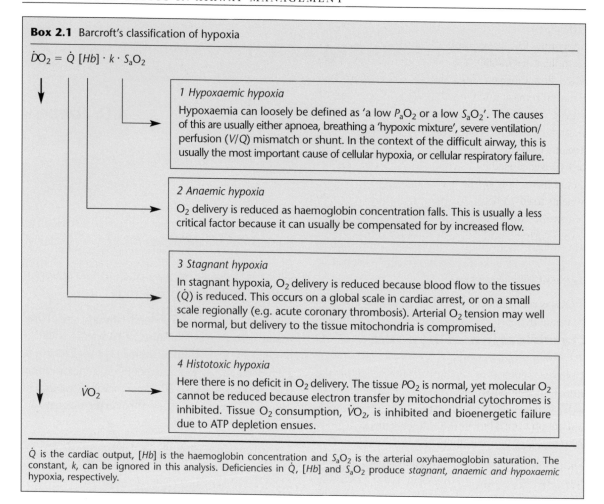

Box 2.1 Barcroft's classification of hypoxia

$$\dot{D}O_2 = \dot{Q}\,[Hb] \cdot k \cdot S_aO_2$$

1 Hypoxaemic hypoxia

Hypoxaemia can loosely be defined as 'a low P_aO_2 or a low S_aO_2'. The causes of this are usually either apnoea, breathing a 'hypoxic mixture', severe ventilation/perfusion (V/Q) mismatch or shunt. In the context of the difficult airway, this is usually the most important cause of cellular hypoxia, or cellular respiratory failure.

2 Anaemic hypoxia

O_2 delivery is reduced as haemoglobin concentration falls. This is usually a less critical factor because it can usually be compensated for by increased flow.

3 Stagnant hypoxia

In stagnant hypoxia, O_2 delivery is reduced because blood flow to the tissues ($\dot{Q}$) is reduced. This occurs on a global scale in cardiac arrest, or on a small scale regionally (e.g. acute coronary thrombosis). Arterial O_2 tension may well be normal, but delivery to the tissue mitochondria is compromised.

4 Histotoxic hypoxia

Here there is no deficit in O_2 delivery. The tissue PO_2 is normal, yet molecular O_2 cannot be reduced because electron transfer by mitochondrial cytochromes is inhibited. Tissue O_2 consumption, $\dot{V}O_2$, is inhibited and bioenergetic failure due to ATP depletion ensues.

$\dot{Q}$ is the cardiac output, $[Hb]$ is the haemoglobin concentration and S_aO_2 is the arterial oxyhaemoglobin saturation. The constant, k, can be ignored in this analysis. Deficiencies in $\dot{Q}$, $[Hb]$ and S_aO_2 produce *stagnant, anaemic and hypoxaemic* hypoxia, respectively.

as a cause of death, since having a haemoglobin concentration of $10\,\mathrm{g\,dl}^{-1}$ is hardly fatal.

Stagnant hypoxia is unlikely to be a cause, since the cardiac output is likely to be elevated as a compensatory mechanism.

The underlying mechanism of cellular death in this case is *histotoxic hypoxia*. Just as carbon monoxide has a high affinity for the haem group in haemoglobin, it also has a high affinity for the iron-containing haem flavoprotein in mitochondrial respiratory cytochromes. Once bound, electron transfer is interrupted and tissue O_2, albeit in abundant supply, cannot be reduced and bioenergetic failure supervenes. In carbon monoxide poisoning, the presence of carboxyhaemoglobin merely serves as a marker of carbon monoxide exposure. It is not usually part of the mechanism of death.

Differential effects of deficits in O_2 delivery

The equation in Box 2.1 shows that $\dot{D}O_2$ is simply proportional to the product of the three 'Barcroft' variables. It would, therefore, appear at first sight that any given deficit in $\dot{D}O_2$ should cause identical degrees of cellular hypoxia regardless of whether the deficit in $\dot{D}O_2$ is due to anaemia, low flow or hypoxaemia. We shall see below that whereas $\dot{D}O_2$ deficits due to anaemic and stagnant hypoxia have virtually identical consequences, $\dot{D}O_2$ deficits due to hypoxaemic hypoxia are very distinct and uniquely important.

Anaemic and stagnant $\dot{D}O_2$ deficits

Experimental and theoretical models show that the variables $[Hb]$ and $\dot{Q}$ are not uniquely independent variables; it is merely the product, $\dot{Q}\,[Hb]$ which determines O_2 delivery and cellular oxygenation. For example, if haemoglobin concentration is halved and blood flow doubled, O_2 delivery and cellular oxygenation remain unchanged. It also follows that the degree of cellular hypoxia caused by a reduction in haemoglobin concentration (while blood flow remains constant) is identical to the degree of cellular hypoxia caused by a proportionally equal reduction in blood flow (while haemoglobin concentration remains fixed). This is because these variables simply determine the flux of O_2 to the tissues, and they have no other significance beyond this point.

Hypoxaemic $\dot{D}O_2$ deficits

If $\dot{D}O_2$ is reduced because of hypoxaemia, the effects on tissue hypoxia are (under certain circumstances) greater than if an equal $\dot{D}O_2$ reduction were due to anaemic or stagnant causes. This seems counterintuitive if considered in terms of Barcroft's classification. This is because Barcroft's classification focuses on O_2 delivery (bulk O_2 flux) to the tissue capillaries, and not on events beyond this; namely transfer of O_2 from capillary to cell and mitochondrion.

While it is true that the term arterial saturation of O_2 (S_aO_2) determines O_2 delivery in the same way as do $\dot{Q}$ and $[Hb]$, it is the P_aO_2 in the capillary which drives the diffusion of O_2 from capillary to cell. So the effects of hypoxaemia are twofold: not only does it reduce O_2 flux along the arterial tree (via a reduced S_aO_2), but it also impairs O_2 delivery beyond the tissue capillary (via a reduced PO_2).

The PO_2 at the cellular level is around 3–10 mmHg, and at the mitochondrion it is around 1 mmHg. The PO_2 in tissue capillaries may be around 40 mmHg and this PO_2 gradient drives O_2 from capillary to mitochondrion according to Fick's law of diffusion. Figure 2.1 shows the effect of reducing $\dot{D}O_2$ on the cell's ability to take-up and consume O_2 ($\dot{V}O_2$), and how this differs depending on whether the fall in $\dot{D}O_2$ is achieved via anaemic/stagnant or hypoxaemic mechanisms. It can be seen that as $\dot{D}O_2$ falls, $\dot{V}O_2$ remains constant until a critical $\dot{D}O_2$, $\dot{D}O_{2crit}$, is reached, below which cellular O_2 uptake and utilization are diminished. $\dot{D}O_{2crit}$ represents the

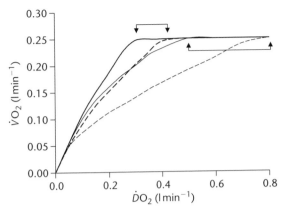

Figure 2.1 Plot of cellular O_2 consumption ($\dot{V}O_2$) vs. bulk O_2 delivery ($\dot{D}O_2$). Solid lines represent stagnant/anaemic hypoxia. Broken lines represent hypoxaemic hypoxia. Bold lines show normal relationship for tissue without significant barrier to O_2 diffusion from capillary to cell. Feint lines represent tissue with significant diffusional resistance, as in oedema or shock. As $\dot{D}O_2$ falls, $\dot{V}O_2$ initially remains constant and satisfies the normal metabolic requirement (0.25 l min^{-1}). When $\dot{D}O_2$ falls to a critical value, $\dot{D}_{crit}$ (shown by arrows), cellular O_2 consumption falls and cellular hypoxia begins. The difference in $\dot{D}_{crit}$ between hypoxaemic and stagnant/anaemic hypoxia is shown to increase when a diffusional barrier exists. Redrawn from Farmery AD, Whiteley JP. A mathematical model of electron transfer within the mitochondrial respiratory cytochromes. *J Theor Biol* 2001; **213**: 197–207.

O_2 delivery at which cellular hypoxia begins. In normal tissue (bold lines), cellular hypoxia is seen to begin when $\dot{D}O_2$ falls to 0.41 min^{-1} for hypoxaemic hypoxia, whereas the cell can tolerate a lower $\dot{D}O_2$ if the mechanism is anaemic or stagnant. In other words, cells are more vulnerable to hypoxaemic hypoxia.

According to Fick's law, diffusive O_2 flux depends not only on the partial pressure gradient, but also on the distance between capillary and cell, and this may be increased in oedematous states (where the interstitium occupies a greater volume, separating capillary from cell), and in capillary de-recruitment due to shock (where, if a cell's nearest capillary is de-recruited, it's new nearest patent capillary will now be a greater distance away). This may explain why the difference between stagnant/anaemic and hypoxaemic hypoxia on cellular O_2 uptake is exaggerated in states of reduced diffusive conductance. This effect is also shown in Figure 2.1 (feint curves).

The rate of arterial desaturation in apnoea

We have seen that hypoxaemic hypoxia is of particular importance in the development of cellular hypoxia and it goes without saying that in the context of the difficult airway, the principal cause of hypoxaemia is airway obstruction. It is important to understand the mechanisms by which hypoxaemia develops, and the factors which determine the rate of this process.

As soon as apnoea (with an obstructed airway) occurs, alveolar and hence pulmonary capillary PO_2 begins to fall. In apnoea, the process of gas exchange between alveolus and pulmonary capillary becomes non-linear. The rising partial pressure of carbon dioxide (PCO_2) and falling pH associated with CO_2 accumulation continually shifts the O_2–haemoglobin dissociation curve adding yet more non-linearity to the process of arterial desaturation. The time lag between changes in PO_2 feeding through into changes in mixed venous PO_2 enhances the complexity of the mathematical model further. Figure 2.2 shows the effects of six different physiological derangements on the rate of arterial desaturation in obstructed apnoea. Figure 2.2(a) shows that desaturation is exaggerated in small lung volumes (as might occur in supine anaesthetized patients). Figure 2.2(b) shows that the value of the initial alveolar O_2 concentration at the onset of apnoea is also important. Due to the various mathematical non-linearities in the system, the lower the initial alveolar O_2 tension, the greater the rate of desaturation. This has important implications for patients who have periods of partial airway obstruction (and hence diminished alveolar PO_2 (P_AO_2)) before obstructing completely. Figure 2.2(c) shows that while shunt diminishes the value of S_aO_2 at any given time during apnoea, the rate of desaturation is unaltered. Figure 2.2(d) shows that increased metabolic rates (as may occur in sepsis, or when struggling to breathe in severe airway obstruction) increases the rate of arterial desaturation, and this effect is exaggerated as desaturation proceeds. Figure 2.2(e) and (f) shows how both diminished cardiac output and reduced haemoglobin concentrations increase the rate of arterial desaturation in apnoea. This is partly because haemoglobin acts as an O_2 reservoir. The effect of cardiac output is complex. This is an interesting finding, because of the effect this will have on O_2 delivery in the Barcroftian sense. So, not only does arterial hypoxaemia have a unique importance in terms of cellular hypoxia (as discussed above and also Figure 2.1), but in apnoea, anaemia and low flow states *compound* the reduction in S_aO_2 and also markedly exaggerate the reduction in O_2 delivery, which is the product of all three of these terms. The interplay of these factors is depicted in Figure 2.3.

Also of note is the fact that small derangements in each of the physiological factors in Figure 2.2 combine to produce a larger overall effect on the rate of arterial desaturation. An example of this might be a 'typical' sick patient about to undergo induction of anaesthesia. This is shown in Figure 2.4.

Hypoxaemia during anaesthesia

Causes of hypoxaemia occurring during anaesthesia can be divided into the following three categories:

1 *Problems with O_2 supply*: This usually involves equipment failure resulting in the delivery of a hypoxic mixture. Meticulous pre-anaesthetic checks, and use of O_2 monitoring at the common gas outlet or in the inspired limb of the breathing system will eliminate this cause.

2 *Problems with O_2 delivery from lips to lung*: The causes of hypoventilation are numerous, but the commonest are central respiratory depression, intrinsic airway obstruction and breathing system obstruction. It is important to note that if patients are breathing high inspired O_2 fractions, hypoxaemia will be a very late (possibly too late) feature of hypoventilation. Figure 2.5 demonstrates how, as alveolar ventilation falls to even very low levels, P_AO_2 is preserved if the inspired O_2 fraction is >30%. This clearly emphasises the fact that pulse oximeters have no place in monitoring the adequacy of ventilation in the critical care setting.

3 *Problems with O_2 transfer from lung to blood*: Under anaesthesia considerable V/Q mismatch occurs. The mechanisms for this are not fully

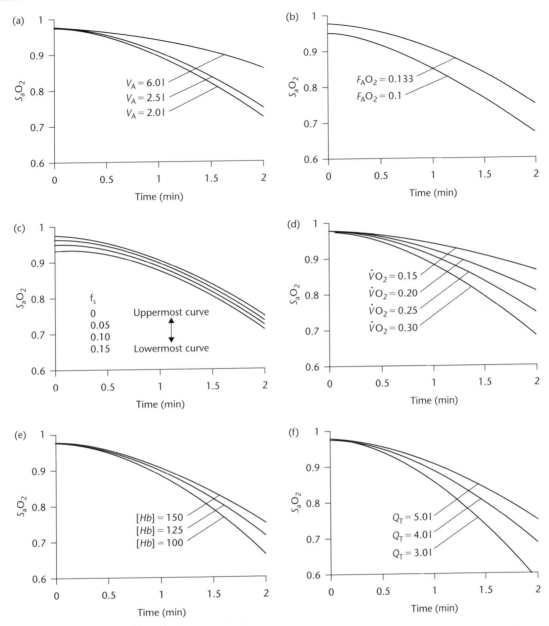

Figure 2.2 (a) Effect of lung volume (V_A in l) on the time course of S_aO_2 in apnoea. (b) Effect of initial F_AO_2 on the time course of S_aO_2 in apnoea. (c) Effect of shunt fraction (f_s) ranging from 0% to 15% on the time course of S_aO_2 in apnoea. (d) Effect of O_2 consumption rate ($\dot{V}O_2$) ranging from 0.15 to 0.3 l min^{-1} on the time course of S_aO_2 in apnoea. (e) Effect of haemoglobin concentration ([Hb] in g l^{-1}) on the time course of S_aO_2 in apnoea. (f) Effect of total blood volume (Q_T) on the time course of S_aO_2 in apnoea. Reproduced with permission from Farmery AD, Roe PG. A model to describe the rate of oxyhaemoglobin desaturation during apnoea. *Br J Anaesth* 1996; **76:** 284–291.

understood but are thought to include inhibition of hypoxic pulmonary vasoconstriction (HPV) by anaesthetic agents. Changes in posture, cephalad movement of the diaphragm and increased thoracic blood volume are also implicated. V/Q mismatching produces hypoxaemia which to a large extent can be restored by increasing the inspired O_2 fraction. This distinguishes it

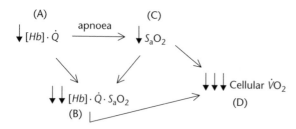

Figure 2.3 Reductions in both [*Hb*] and $\dot{Q}$ as shown in (A) not only reduce O_2 delivery (B) directly (path A–B), but also indirectly via path (A–C–B) during apnoea because the rate of arterial desaturation during apnoea is increased by anaemia and low output. The combination of this direct and indirect effect is to produce an exaggerated reduction in O_2 delivery (B). The reduction in O_2 delivery may reduce cellular O_2 uptake (path B–D), as predicted by the solid lines in Figure 2.1. In addition, the hypoxaemic conditions (point C) contribute independently to exaggerating the reduction of cellular O_2 uptake (via path C–D) as predicted by the broken lines in Figure 2.1.

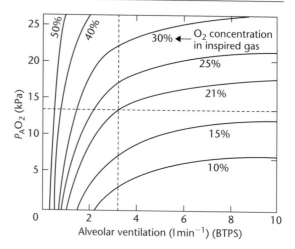

Figure 2.5 Relationship between F_iO_2, alveolar ventilation and P_AO_2.

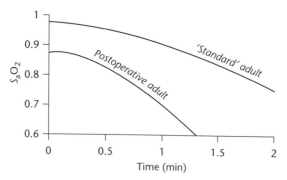

Figure 2.4 Rate of arterial oxyhaemoglobin desaturation with combination of small derangements in pathophysiological variables as might be seen in a perioperative adult. Haemoglobin = 10 g dl^{-1}, cardiac output = 4 l min^{-1}, initial P_AO_2 = 10 kPa, initial P_ACO_2 = 8 kPa, alveolar volume = 2.0 l, shunt fraction (f_s) = 0.1. Reproduced with permission from Farmery AD, Roe PG. A model to describe the rate of oxyhaemoglobin desaturation during apnoea. *Br J Anaesth* 1996; **76**: 284–291.

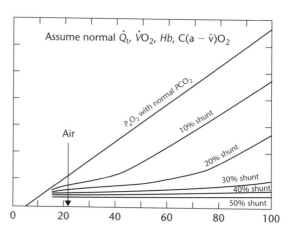

Figure 2.6 Effect of changes in inspired O_2 concentration on P_aO_2 for various right-to-left transpulmonary true shunts. Cardiac output, haemoglobin, O_2 consumption and arteriovenous O_2 content differences were assumed to be normal. Reproduced with permission from Nunn JF. *Applied Respiratory Physiology*, 3rd edition. Butterworths, 1987.

from shunt. 'Shunt' is a term used to describe regions of lung with perfusion but no ventilation as may occur in acute respiratory distress syndrome (ARDS) or pneumonia. Increasing the inspired O_2 fraction has little effect on oxygenation here if the shunt fraction (f_s) is >30%. Oxygenation can often be improved in shunt

and V/Q abnormalities by increasing the cardiac output (increasing cardiac output may result in perfusion of ventilated areas of lung as well as increasing O_2 flux which will increase the mixed venous PO_2 and diminish the effect of the shunt), and application of positive end-expiratory pressure (PEEP) or continuous positive airway pressure (CPAP) to recruit more alveoli.

Causes of hypoventilation	Causes of V/Q mismatch
Obstructed airway	Anaesthesia
Pneumothorax	Bronchial intubation
Obstructed tube/breathing system, defective ventilator	Oesophageal intubation
	Aspiration
Central respiratory depression	Lung disease
	Embolism
Peripheral weakness	

Pre-oxygenation

Pre-oxygenation aims to increase body O_2 stores to their maximum, so that periods of apnoea are tolerated for longer before critical desaturation occurs. There are two elements within the practice of pre-oxygenation:

- *Supplying 100% inspired O_2*: Good pre-oxygenation technique involves a close-fitting face mask so that the patient breathes the delivered fresh gas rather than entraining air around the mask. Correct face mask application can be confirmed by seeing a full reservoir bag which moves with respiration. The bag is an essential component of the circuit because it provides the reservoir necessary when the patient's peak inspiratory flow ($\sim 30\,l\,min^{-1}$) exceeds the fresh gas flow. The fresh gas flow should be high enough to prevent any rebreathing within the circuit, a problem with the Bain circuit particularly. The circle absorber system is much less affected by rebreathing but the circuit itself has a high volume which may be filled with air initially. It is reasonable, therefore, to pre-oxygenate always with maximal inflow of O_2 into the circuit, preferably at least $10\,l\,min^{-1}$. If the inspired O_2 is <100%, the time to critical desaturation will be reduced.
- *Time required for effective de-nitrogenation with 100% O_2*: The aim is to maximize O_2 stores within the lung and the blood. The blood stores of O_2 do *not* change dramatically with pre-oxygenation. If the haemoglobin is 98% saturated on room air and rises to 100% with pre-oxygenation, then the increase is minimal. The amount of O_2 dissolved

in the plasma is increased by the rise in partial pressure, but this is trivial.

O_2 content of blood

- O_2 carried by Hb = [*Hb*] conc $\times$ saturation $\times$ 1.39 ml 100 ml^{-1} blood

- O_2 dissolved in plasma = O_2 partial pressure (kPa) $\times$ 0.022 ml 100 ml^{-1} plasma

---

The major change during pre-oxygenation is in the amount of O_2 in the lungs. At the end of a quiet expiration the lung volume at functional residual capacity (FRC) is normally about 2500 ml. This will be affected by patient position or disease processes and may be much reduced by obesity, pregnancy or a distended bowel. On breathing 100% O_2, the wash-in of O_2 is exponential. The time constant (τ) of this wash-in process is the ratio of FRC or alveolar volume to alveolar ventilation ($V_A / \dot{V}_A$). Given an alveolar minute ventilation of $4\,l\,min^{-1}$ and FRC volume of $2.5\,l$ we can estimate the time constant to be $2.5/4 = 0.625\,min$. After 3 time constants ($1.9\,min$), the exponential process will be 95% complete.

Exponential wash-in of O_2 during pre-oxygenation (typical values)

- Time constant (*t*) of exponential process = $V_A / \dot{V}_A$ = 2.5/4 = 0.63 min
- After 1 time constant (0.63 min) pre-oxygenation in 37% complete
- After 2 time constants (1.25 min) pre-oxygenation is 68% complete
- After 3 time constants (1.9 min) pre-oxygenation is 95% complete

---

It is, therefore, reasonable to continue pre-oxygenation for at least 3 time constants to ensure maximal pre-oxygenation. It should be noted that patients with a small FRC will pre-oxygenate more quickly than normal but the O_2 store contained in the FRC will be reduced. Increasing alveolar minute ventilation (4–8 deep or vital capacity breaths) increases the rapidity of increase in P_AO_2 and is extremely useful when time for pre-oxygenation is limited. Administering opioids such as fentanyl before pre-oxygenation may lengthen the time required to achieve a high P_AO_2.

In any particular patient, the magnitude of the alveolar minute ventilation and FRC are unknown. It is, therefore, useful to monitor the process of de-nitrogenation by measuring end-tidal FO_2. An end-tidal FO_2 of 90–91% indicates maximal pre-oxygenation and a store of O_2 in the FRC of >2000 ml. In order to use the end-tidal O_2 to guide pre-oxygenation, gas sampling must be reliable (tight-fitting face mask) and gas should not have bi-directional flow over the capnograph sampling line (use a circle absorber circuit not a Bain system). The overall increase in O_2 stores in the blood and lungs with pre-oxygenation is from 1200 ml (air) to 3500 ml.

Desaturation following the use of succinylcholine

The American Society of Anesthesiologists (ASA) difficult airway algorithm recommends that if initial attempts at tracheal intubation after the induction

of general anaesthesia are unsuccessful, the anaesthetist should 'consider the advisability of awakening the patient'. 'Awakening' more realistically means allowing return to an unparalysed state that permits spontaneous ventilation. This is considered to be safe practice. However, to what level might arterial saturation fall before spontaneous ventilation resumes? Using a combination of clinical data and a theoretical model, Benumof demonstrated that during complete obstructive apnoea, and in the 'can't intubate, can't ventilate' situation, critical haemoglobin desaturation occurs before the time to functional recovery for various patients receiving $1\,mg\,kg^{-1}$ of intravenous succinylcholine.

Figure 2.7 shows that in all but the 'normal' adult, critical desaturation occurs long before recovery of even 10% of neuromuscular function.

From this analysis it is clear that in a complete 'can't ventilate, can't intubate' situation, it is not appropriate to wait for the return of spontaneous ventilation, but rather a rescue option should be pursued immediately. Benumof points out that this analysis ignores the central respiratory depressant effects of the concomitantly administered general anaesthetics, and so this should be regarded as an underestimation of the time to functional recovery.

Time to haemoglobin desaturation with initial $F_AO_2 = 0.87$

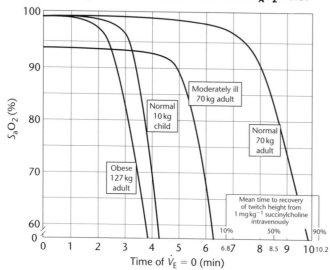

Figure 2.7 S_aO_2 vs. time of apnoea for various types of patients. Reproduced with permission from Benumof JL, Dagg R, Benumof R. Critical haemoglobin desaturation will occur before return to an unparalyzed state following 1 mg/kg intravenous succinylcholine. *Anesthesiology* 1997; **87**: 979–982.

The final common pathway of cellular hypoxia: membrane potential and cell death

Venous PO_2 is a reasonable indicator of *capillary* and hence *tissue* PO_2. In many respects, measuring venous PO_2 (either mixed venous, or organ specific venous such as jugular venous) is more useful in evaluating tissue oxygenation than measuring P_aO_2. Experimental and clinical evidence suggests that consciousness is lost when jugular venous PO_2 (and hence 'tissue PO_2' in the watershed of this drainage) falls below 20 mmHg. It is this PO_2 which drives diffusion of O_2 to its final destination in the mitochondria, where the PO_2 may be a fraction of a mmHg. With this degree of mitochondrial hypoxia, electron transfer cannot proceed (there is insufficient available molecular O_2 to accept electrons). This redox reaction falters and there is insufficient energy production to power the generation of ATP. We discuss the events which follow the onset of cellular bioenergetic failure.

Tissues vary in their sensitivity to hypoxia, but cortical neurones are particularly sensitive. They (along with the myocardium) are perhaps the most clinically important and are therefore the most studied. It is said that 'hypoxia stops the machine and wrecks the machinery'. As far as neurones and the myocardium are concerned this aphorism means that hypoxia initially arrests cellular function. For a period of time the integrity of the cell and its viability remain intact. If hypoxia is reversed, function will resume. However, sustained hypoxia wrecks the machinery. Via numerous and complex mechanisms, and in neurones particularly, an accelerating series of destructive events ensues, which result in cell death. The length of this process is highly variable depending on the tissue, the metabolic rate, blood flow and many other factors. However, it may be as short as 4 min for some neurones.

Anoxia and membrane potential

In general, living cells can be characterized by possession of a resting membrane potential whereas dead cells have no resting membrane potential. The effect of anoxia on resting membrane potential depends on the nature of the anoxic insult. In ischaemia (as in stroke), the tissue is deprived of O_2 and blood flow, whereas in airway obstruction, hypoxaemia occurs while blood flow (and glucose supply) continues, and this may have more deleterious effects.

One of the first metabolic features of mitochondrial bioenergetic failure is the depletion in ATP and accumulation of NADH. Small amounts of ATP can be generated from the glycolytic pathway, but this requires oxidized nicotinamide adenine dinucleotide (NAD^+) which is in short supply. However, the necessary NAD^+ can be generated by converting pyruvate to lactate, thus facilitating limited ATP production anaerobically. The intracellular acidosis which results from anaerobic metabolism is one of the first changes to be detected following cellular anoxia. If the nature of the hypoxia is *hypoxaemic hypoxia*, then blood flow will be preserved and there will be an abundant supply of glucose which will exacerbate the acidosis. Hyperglycaemic patients are particularly at risk.

Shortly after the onset of intracellular acidosis, the membrane potential of neurones begins to change. This is shown in Figure 2.8. The effect is variable, but the majority hyperpolarize. It is thought that this is due to an increase in K^+ channel conductance. The mechanisms are not clear but possibilities include activation of ATP-sensitive K^+ channels (increased conductance in low ATP states), activation of direct O_2-sensitive K^+ channels or activation of pH-sensitive K^+ channels. Hyperpolarization of neurones renders them less susceptible to synaptic activation, and this may manifest as loss of consciousness (i.e. 'the machine stops').

From this point, membrane potential changes from hyperpolarization to slow depolarization. The mechanism of this is thought to be that the increased K^+ conductance (which initially hyperpolarized the membrane) allows K^+ efflux out of the cell down its concentration gradient. This escaped K^+ is normally removed from the extracellular space by the Na^+–K^+-ATPase, but as this pump begins to fail, extracellular $[K^+]$ increases and, as can be predicted by the Nernst equation, resting membrane potential

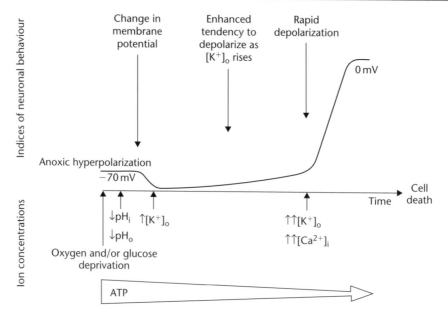

Figure 2.8 Membrane potential changes induced by cellular hypoxia. Intra- and extracellular pH changes are the first to be observed. Changes in membrane potential occur between 15 and 90 s. This is usually hyperpolarization due to increased K^+ channel conductance. K^+ then leaks from within the cell. This causes an increase in extracellular $[K^+]$, especially if perfusion is limited (as in ischaemia), since the extracellular space is not washed-out of ions and metabolites. The increasing extracellular $[K^+]$ causes gradual membrane depolarization which in turn activates voltage-sensitive Ca^{2+} channels, contributing further to the depolarization. The increasing acidosis and increasing depolarization triggers Ca^{2+} release from intracellular stores, which in turn triggers synaptic release of glutamate. The release of this massive amount of glutamate stimulates ligand-gated cation channels whose opening coincides with a very rapid phase of membrane depolarization. At this point, the Na^+–K^+–ATPase pump has ceased to operate and membrane potential is lost irretrievably.

begins to depolarize. As the membrane potential depolarizes further, Ca^{2+} channels are activated and Ca^{2+} influx contributes to an acceleration of the depolarization.

At this point, these electrophysiological effects are reversible if oxygenation is restored. If not, a cascade of irreversible events ensues.

Within a short time, membrane depolarization becomes very rapid. This coincides with a number of cellular events: the failure of the Na^+–K^+–ATPase pump, massive release of Ca^{2+} from intracellular stores triggering massive release of excitatory neurotransmitters (principally glutamate) from synaptic vesicles, which in turn stimulate glutamate receptor-linked ion channels triggering further cation influx into the cell. Beyond this point, cell survival is unlikely. The machine is wrecked.

The time course for these events is variable. It is quickest for neurones exposed to ischaemia (arrested flow) under hyperglycaemic and hyperthermic conditions, where the process may be a matter of only 1–4 min. Under hypoxaemic conditions with preserved flow and normoglycaemia, the process may take between 4 and 15 min depending on the degree and abruptness of the insult.

Key points

- Tissue hypoxia can be fatal despite normoxaemia (cyanide and CO poisoning).
- Hypoxaemic hypoxia (airway obstruction) is more damaging to cells than anaemic or stagnant hypoxia.
- Oximeters measure saturation not ventilation. A normal saturation does not mean that ventilation is not dangerously depressed.

- Oxygen saturation will fall more quickly in an apnoeic sick patient. Waiting for spontaneous ventilation to return may not be a sensible option.
- An end-tidal oxygen of >90% indicates maximum preoxygenation.
- Preoxygenation achieves its end by increasing the amount of oxygen in the lung.

Further reading

Farmery AD, Roe PG. A model to describe the rate of oxyhaemoglobin desaturation during apnoea. *Br J Anaesth* 1996; **76**: 284–291.

Farmery AD, Whiteley JP. A mathematical model of electron transfer within the mitochondrial respiratory cytochromes. *J Theor Biol* 2001; **213**: 197–207.

Benumof JL, Dagg R, Benumof R. Critical hemoglobin desaturation will occur before return to an unparalyzed state following 1 mg/kg intravenous succinylcholine. *Anesthesiology* 1997; **87**: 979–982.

Benumof JL. Preoxygenation. *Anesthesiology* 1999; **91**: 603–605.

PHYSICS AND PHYSIOLOGY

3

A.D. Farmery

Physics of airflow

Gas flowing through tubes can be characterized by possessing either *laminar* or *turbulent* flow, or more usually, a mixture of both. Before we explore these, we need to familiarize ourselves with a fundamental thermodynamic concept detailed below.

BOX 3.1

- Flowing particles of gas possess ENERGY.
- This can be in the form of *potential energy* (i.e. its pressure, P) or in the form of kinetic energy, due to its velocity ($1/2\, \rho v^2$).
- If no energy is lost from the system then the sum of these two forms of energy is constant.

$$P + \frac{1}{2}\rho v^2 = \text{total energy (constant)}$$

↗ ↖ Bernouilli's principle
potential energy   kinetic energy

Laminar flow

In laminar flow, although gas molecules in different parts of the 'stream' have different velocities, the vectors of these velocities are parallel, as shown in Figure 3.1.

For a viscous Newtonian fluid such as air, molecules can be thought of as being arranged in slippery

'sheets' or 'layers' and these have been schematically labelled 1, 2, 3, etc. in Figure 3.1. The sheet of molecules closest to the wall of the tube (sheet 1) is stationary and bound to the wall of the tube. Each sheet of molecules can exert a force on its neighbour ('shear' force) so that a slow moving sheet will tend to retard a quicker moving neighbour, and quicker moving sheets will tend to drag slower neighbours along. For example, the shear forces exerted on sheet 2 by the stationary sheet 1 would tend to retard it, but the shear force exerted by its other neighbour, the faster moving sheet 3, would tend to increase its velocity. The sheets of molecules in the middle of the stream (e.g. sheet 3) are the least influenced by the static layers at the edges, and so these have the highest velocity. The amount of grip which one sheet has on another (the shear force) is a property of the *viscosity* of the fluid. For low viscosity (i.e. slippery) fluids, the stationary boundary layer has little 'grip' on its neighbour and so the velocity of subsequent layers rises very quickly as one moves towards the centre of the stream. For high viscosity (sticky) fluids the stationary boundary layer grips its neighbour and retards it. This layer, in turn, retards the next innermost layer, and so on. The result is that successive layers increase in velocity towards the centre only slowly.

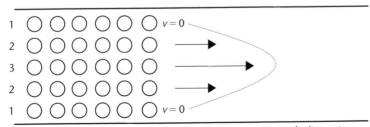

Numbers represent 'layers' of molecules. Arrows represent velocity vectors.

Figure 3.1 Laminar flow.

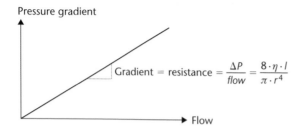

Figure 3.2 Pressure gradient versus flow diagram.

1 *'Pressure-drop' and 'flow' are linearly related in laminar flow*

For laminar flow, pressure and flow are analogous to electrical voltage and current. The relationship is described by Poiseuille's law, which is analogous to Ohm's law, and is shown in Figure 3.2.

For a gas moving in a tube such as shown in Figure 3.1, the friction (or shear forces) created as layers slide over each other, will generate heat and so energy will be lost from the gas as it passes down the tube (energy lost = mean friction force × distance down the tube). Given that the mean friction force is constant at any point along the tube, there must be a constant (or linear) loss of energy with distance travelled down the tube. What effect will this have on the gas pressure down the tube?

From the equation in Box 3.1, the 'kinetic term' must be constant, because the mean velocity of the layers of molecules is the same at any point along the tube. So by deduction, this must mean that the linear drop in energy (as heat is liberated by friction as the gas flows down the tube) must be manifest as a linear drop in *pressure* along the tube. This explains the obedience to Ohm's/Poiseuille's law as shown in Figure 3.2.

The key feature of laminar flow is that the velocity vectors of all the sheets are parallel and although each layer has a different velocity to its neighbour, each sheet retains its own velocity and so there is no change in the relative velocities, and the *mean* velocity at any point remains constant. Laminar flow is favoured for viscous fluids at low velocities in long narrow tubes with smooth sides. These properties

are quantified by the Reynold's number, N_R, which is given by:

$$N_R = \frac{\rho \cdot \bar{V} \cdot D}{\mu \cdot g}$$

where ρ is density, $\bar{V}$ is mean linear velocity, D is pipe diameter, μ is viscosity and g is a gravitational factor.

For Reynold's numbers below 2000, laminar flow is favoured and above 2000 turbulent flow dominates.

Turbulent flow

In turbulent flow, molecules do not move as sheets slipping over each other with parallel velocity vectors in such an orderly way, but rather swirl and eddy in a seemingly random way. So in turbulent flow, molecules not only have a linear velocity down the length of the pipe, but also a turbulent or rotational velocity as they swirl around in eddies and vortices (Figure 3.3).

1 *'Pressure-drop' and 'flow' have a quadratic relationship in turbulent flow*

Turbulent kinetic energy (due to the velocity of molecules swirling round eddies) amounts to a few percent of the linear kinetic energy, and is a fixed proportion of it. As these molecules swirl around, their turbulent kinetic energy is dissipated as they collide with each other and the pipe wall, and so energy is lost at a greater rate than compared to laminar flow. The rate at which energy is lost is proportional to the turbulent kinetic energy which the molecules possess and this in turn is proportional to the mean linear kinetic energy (Figure 3.4). This energy loss is 'paid for' by a drop in static pressure. The above can be summarized as follows:

ΔP = energy dissipated ∝ turbulent kinetic energy ∝ linear kinetic enery ∝ $\rho \cdot$ flow^2

The relative importance of *viscosity* and *density* in *upper* and *lower* airway obstruction

Acute bronchospasm is characterized by narrowing, due to bronchial smooth muscle contraction

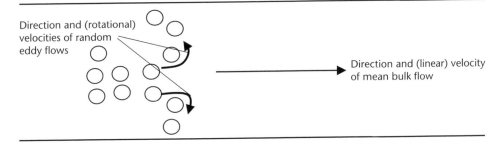

Figure 3.3 Turbulent flow.

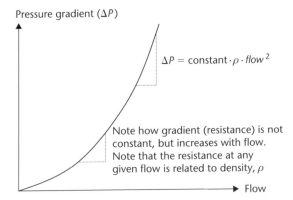

Figure 3.4 Turbulent kinetic energy.

and mucosal inflammation, of the distal airways. This process occurs to some extent throughout the bronchial tree, but its effect on small distal airways has the biggest contribution to the increased airways resistance. This can be appreciated by considering the Poiseuille equation:

$$\text{Resistance } (R) \propto 1/r^4$$

From this we see that the *change* in resistance, R, per unit change in airway radius, r (dR/dr) is proportional to $1/r^5$. In other words, the smaller the airway, the greater will be the increase in resistance resulting from a further reduction in radius.

1 *Is it possible to increase airflow in acute bronchospasm by giving a low density gas such as Heliox?*
The total cross-sectional area of the 11th generation of the bronchial tree is believed to be about seven times larger than at the lobar bronchi, so that flow is characteristically laminar. In this region molecules move as orderly sheets sliding over each other and the friction between these

sheets, which is responsible for the energy loss and pressure drop, is a function of the *viscosity* of the gas and not its *density*. So reducing the density of the gas will have no effect on the pressure gradient required to achieve the same flow. Heliox at 70%/30% (helium/oxygen) is about one-fifth of the density of 70%/30% (nitrogen/oxygen), but its *viscosity* is about the same. For this reason, its use makes little difference to *total* airways resistance because the site of predominant resistance is the small airways where laminar flow predominates. However, turbulence may occur in acute asthma, where the entire bronchial tree may be affected. Whether Heliox is helpful is debated, but a recent review concluded that there is some evidence of benefit, particularly in severe cases.

2 *Is Heliox useful in upper airway obstruction?*
Wherever turbulent flow prevails, the flow for a given pressure gradient is a function of the *density* of the gas. This is because the kinetic energy lost as molecules whiz around eddies is a property of their speed and mass (i.e. density), rather than their 'stickiness'. So if the site of maximum airways resistance is a site at which turbulent flow occurs, then using Heliox will greatly increase flow for a given pressure gradient, or allow the same flow for a smaller pressure gradient. Clinical examples of this include:

- upper airway obstruction from haematoma, tissue swelling or tumour;
- laryngeal obstruction from oedema/infection, nerve palsy, tumour;
- large airway obstruction from tumour or extrinsic vascular compression.

The benefits of Heliox however are double-edged. The higher the concentration of helium in the mixture, the lower, by definition, will be the F_iO_2. For most patients with critical airflow obstruction, the decision to give any gas other than 100% oxygen (O_2) needs to be made very carefully. It would be difficult to justify giving nitrous oxide, which has a higher density than O_2.

Physics of distensible airways

Anatomy

The anatomy of the upper airway is depicted in Figure 3.5. The nasopharynx is a rigid bony structure and is therefore not liable to collapse. Likewise the trachea, with its supporting cartilaginous structure is rigid and resistant to collapse. However, the intervening segment, the pharynx, is not supported by bone or cartilage and is therefore potentially collapsible. In adults, the commonest site for airway collapse in sleep and anaesthesia is the velopharynx (where the soft palate meets the posterior pharyngeal wall). This has been shown in radiological studies during both inhalational and intravenous anaesthesia. This contradicts the previously commonly held view that the principal site of airway obstruction was retrolingual, and caused by posterior displacement of the tongue. In one study of isoflurane anaesthesia, retrolingual obstruction accounted for only 2 of 16 subjects, the remaining obstructed at the level of the velopharynx and larynx.

The Starling resistor

The *functional* anatomy of the upper airway can be reduced to a consideration of a collapsible segment (the pharynx) between two rigid segments (the nasopharynx and the trachea) as shown in Figure 3.6. This system behaves as a 'Starling resistor' and airflow can become limited or completely abolished during spontaneous ('negative intrathoracic pressure') breathing as described below. A Starling resistor is one whose characteristics can be ohmic (i.e. flow is simply dependent of the difference between upstream pressure, P_u, and downstream pressures, P_d) under certain conditions, and non-ohmic under

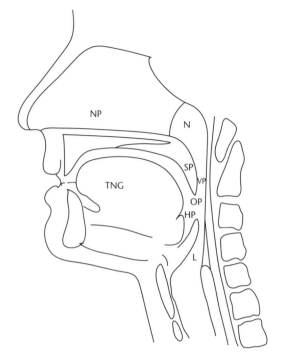

Figure 3.5 Anatomy of the upper airway. NP: nasopharynx; TNG: tongue; SP: soft palate; VP: velopharynx; OP: oropharynx; HP: hypopharynx; L: larynx.

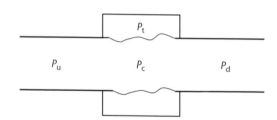

Figure 3.6 Functional anatomy of the upper airway between the segments. P_t: tissue pressure; P_u: upstream pressure; P_d: downstream pressure; P_c: pressure at site of collapsible segment.

other circumstances (when flow becomes independent of downstream pressure, yet dependent on transmural pressure at the site of the distensible segment).

The value of Pressure at the site of a collapsible segment (P_c) lies somewhere between P_u and P_d, tending towards P_u at the upstream end and P_d at the downstream end. This resistor can exist in one of the three states as depicted in Figure 3.7.

The Starling resistor is analogous to water flowing over a weir where the heights of the upstream and

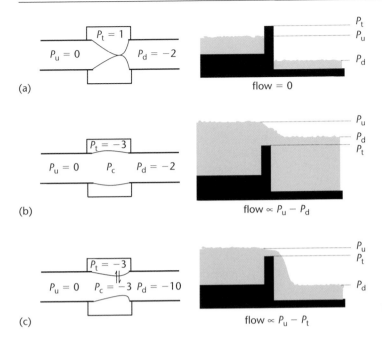

Figure 3.7 Three states in a Starling resistor.

downstream sections are analogous to P_u and P_d, and the height of the weir is analogous to tissue pressure (P_t). This is shown is Figure 3.7.

Figure 3.7 shows that

(a) When P_t always exceeds P_u, P_c and P_d, the distensible segment will move inwards and occlude the airway completely. Here flow = 0.

(b) When P_u, P_c and P_d always exceed P_t, the distensible segment will always be open and the tube behaves as simple ohmic resistor where flow $\propto (P_u - P_d)$.

(c) When $P_u > P_t > P_d$, the airway remains patent at its upstream end (where P_c is close to P_u and greater than P_t) and tends to partially collapse at its downstream end where P_c tends to P_d. Here flow is proportional to $(P_u - P_t)$ rather than $(P_u - P_d)$. Note how flow over the weir cannot be increased by merely lowering the height of the downstream weir-pool.

Similarly in the upper airway under these conditions, flow cannot be increased by lowering P_d (i.e. by increasing inspiratory effort) because by doing so the distensible segment moves further in, thus buffering the effect of this drop in P_d at the site of

the constriction, so that P_c remains in equilibrium with P_t and hence remains constant. As flow is proportional to $P_u - P_t$, it too remains constant despite increasing inspiratory effort. In this state flow can only be increased by increasing upstream pressure with, for example, continous positive airway pressure (CPAP).

Critical instability at points of narrowing

Points of narrowing within the upper airway such as enlarged tonsils or partial posterior displacement of the tongue can potentially lead to critical instability in upper airway patency. Consider a narrowing such as shown in Figure 3.7c. Here the airway wall has moved inwards until the pressure at the site of constriction has equilibrated with the tissue pressure, thus buffering the fall in P_c which would have otherwise resulted from the lowering of P_d. However, this has created a constriction at this site with a resultant force increase in the velocity of the gas at this point. According to Bernoulli's principle (Box 3.1) this will result in a fall in pressure P_c which will be buffered to some extent by further inward movement of the airway wall. This unstable cycle repeats itself until collapse occurs.

Obstructed

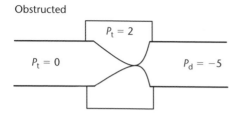

Post-cricothyrotomy

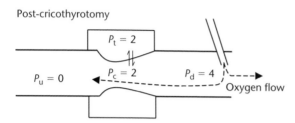

Figure 3.8 Properties of Starling resistor.

Needle cricothyrotomy

In the event of complete airway collapse despite attempted application of CPAP or positive pressure mask ventilation, oxygenation can be facilitated via a needle cricothyrotomy. Reasonable 'tidal volumes' of O_2 can be passed via a relatively fine bore needle because we are able to apply great driving pressure either via a bag or direct intermittent connection to the wall-mounted rotameter. However, there is a theoretical risk that since the upper airway is obstructed, gas may not be able to leave the lungs resulting in dangerous hyperinflation.

Figure 3.8 shows how, due to the properties of a Starling resistor, this risk is small and mostly unrealised.

Passage of O_2 into the trachea, downstream of the obstruction, increases P_d such that it now exceeds P_t. Excess gas can now easily escape without risk of hyperinflation. With the airway now partially open, application of CPAP via a face mask may now aid convection and diffusion of O_2 down the trachea, and excess retrograde O_2 leak (from the cricothyrotomy site to the upper airway) can be controlled.

Flow-volume loops

We will restrict our discussions to analysis of flow-volume (FV) loops seen in *extrathoracic* airway obstruction, as opposed to the more familiar FV

loops seen in intrathoracic airway obstruction, such as asthma and emphysema. Extrathoracic obstructions are classified in Box 3.2.

Box 3.2

Extrathoracic airway obstruction: classification

- Fixed obstruction:
  - tumour in larynx or main bronchus
  - tracheal stenosis; post-tracheostomy
  - laryngeal tumour, oedema, paresis
  - aspirated foreign body.

- Variable airway obstruction:
  - distensible collapsible airway (Starling resistor)
  - distensible collapsible airway with constriction point:
    - tonsilar hyperplasia
    - posterior movement of tongues
  - 'flap-valve' effect from foreign body.

FV loop patterns for extrathoracic airway obstruction are distinctive, and furthermore, fixed and variable obstructions can also be distinguished. Figure 3.9 shows these patterns for fixed and variable extrathoracic obstructions compared with a normal FV loop.

Normal FV loops are characterized by the rapid emptying of the lung from total lung capacity (TLC); peak-flow being achieved early in the breath. Thereafter there is a linear decay in flow as the lung empties (the so-called 'effort independent' part of the loop). The inspiratory limb is almost 'semi-circular'.

Fixed extrathoracic obstructions produce a FV loop whose inspiratory and expiratory limbs are almost symmetrical. The loop is more 'box-like' than 'loop-like' on account of the maximum inspiratory and expiratory flows being held constant for most of the breath duration.

What physical properties of the lung account for these differences in the FV loop? To understand this we need to consider some lung-mechanics for normal airway emptying. Figure 3.10 shows pressures at various points in the airway during expiration. During breath-holding (Figure 3.10a) with an open glottis there is no flow and pressure = 0 (atmospheric) at all points. Note how the intrapleural pressure is sub-atmospheric ($-7\,cmH_2O$) as this pressure

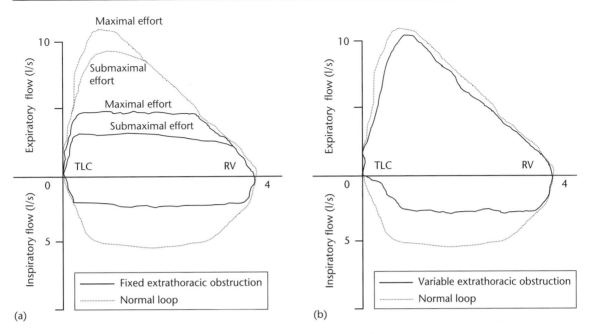

Figure 3.9 FV loop patterns for extrathoracic airway obstruction.

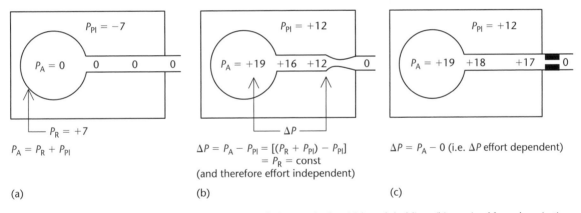

Figure 3.10 Pressures at various points in the airway during expiration (a) breath holding, (b) maximal forced-expiration: normal lung mechanics, (c) maximal forced-expiration: extrathoracic obstruction.

must equal and oppose the recoil pressure of the lung ($+7\,cmH_2O$) which would tend to collapse the lung. The alveolar pressure therefore always exceeds pleural pressure by an amount equal to the recoil pressure ($P_A = P_{Pl} + P_R$).

During maximal forced expiration (Figure 3.10b) if the pleural pressure is raised say to $12\,cmH_2O$, then the alveolar pressure will equal $19\,cmH_2O$ and flow will occur along the airway. Flow through the airway resistance causes pressure to drop along its passage until at a certain point (the 'equal pressure point' or

EPP) the intraluminal pressure equals the pleural pressure which in this example is $12\,cmH_2O$. At this point, for the first time, transmural pressure becomes positive and causes airway narrowing. This narrowing causes airflow to accelerate and approach the critical wave speed (i.e. the speed of sound). So beyond this point, gas travels at a higher velocity than the speed at which pressure waves can travel. This being the case, the downstream pressure caused by (or causing) this airflow cannot be transmitted upstream and so *downstream* pressure can have no influence on it. Therefore the only influence on airflow is the 'pressure gradient' ΔP, *upstream* of the EPP which equals $19 - 12 = 7\,cmH_2O$. In other words, the driving pressure for airflow, ΔP, is simply equal to the recoil pressure which is a *constant*. It therefore follows that airflow will reach a maximal value which is uninfluenced by expiratory effort. The only reason flow decays throughout the breath is that as the lung empties and gets smaller, the calibre of the airways also gets smaller and so flow falls in proportion to lung *volume* and not *effort*. This lack of effort dependency is demonstrated by the fact that the maximal and submaximal dotted curves share the same envelope for most of the latter part of the breath.

In extrathoracic airway obstruction (Figure 3.10c), no equal pressure point within the intrathoracic airways exists because the site of maximal airflow limitation is the *extrathoracic* resistance. Upstream of this, intraluminal pressure always exceeds the intrapleural pressure and so the driving pressure to flow, ΔP, is simply the alveolar pressure, P_A and hence it is 'effort-dependent'. This is evidenced by the fact that the maximal and submaximal expiratory curves have distinctly different envelopes.

Because the intraluminal pressure always exceeds the intrapleural pressure, the tendency for the airway calibre to reduce as the lung gets smaller is reduced (*c.f.* the normal situation). For this reason, although flow is dependent on effort, it is independent of lung volume, and this accounts for the long flat plateau in the expiratory curve.

Variable vs. fixed obstruction

Figure 3.9b shows a FV loop in variable obstruction as may occur during sleep, and following anaesthesia without necessarily any airway pathology. The dominant characteristic of this loop is that expiration is essentially normal, whereas inspiration is markedly impaired for reasons discussed in Section 2.2.

Physiology of the upper airway

In Section 2.2, we discussed the physical properties of flow in collapsible tubes and the propensity for airway collapse or flow-limitation as the airway adopts the characteristics of a Starling resistor. Clearly this property is not ideal, and so it is not surprising that physiological mechanisms exist to minimize such airflow disturbance. Such mechanisms involve the co-ordinated activation of muscle groups which oppose airway collapse.

Muscle groups of the upper airway

There are more than 20 muscles surrounding the upper airway which constrict and dilate its lumen. For simplicity we shall lump these together as 'pharyngeal dilator muscles', but in reality these groups of muscles interact to determine the patency of the airway in a complex fashion which is not fully understood. The most widely studied of these muscles is genioglossus, which principally controls the position of the tongue and hyoid apparatus.

An important bony structure that determines the airway size is the mandible, to which muscle and soft tissue are attached. It can therefore act as a lever and tensor.

It is thought unlikely that the pharynx is dilated by active dilatation on muscle groups within the pharyngeal wall, but rather paradoxically that these muscles actively *constrict*. Evidence for this is provided by the fact that the electromyographic (EMG) activity of these muscles *increases* as the pharynx dilates. It remains unclear whether the 'dilator' muscles act to dilate the airway, or whether the increase in muscle tone merely acts to stabilize the airway to withstand the collapsing forces present during inspiration.

Control of pharyngeal dilator activity

The activity of the pharyngeal dilator muscles is influenced by many factors, including arterial PO_2 and PCO_2, airway PCO_2, arousal, hormones (progesterone/oestrogen), lung volume and intrapharyngeal negative pressure.

- *Local reflexes*: The upper airway is richly supplied with receptors, including baroreceptors and chemoreceptors which play a role in modulating the baseline steady-state (i.e. tonic) EMG activity of pharyngeal dilators. Airway baroreceptors detect any fall in upper airway pressure and, possibly via a centrally mediated reflex, increase muscle tone to oppose the airway collapse which such a negative pressure would otherwise have produced. The tonic EMG activity is reduced if this reflex is blocked by application of local anaesthesia to the upper airway. Similarly, EMG activity is reduced when patients switch between breathing via the upper airway and breathing via a tracheostomy.

- *Phasic and central pharyngeal muscle activity*: In addition to the background or 'tonic' activity, pharyngeal muscles also have 'phasic' activity, that is, their EMG activity occurs in phase with tidal ventilation: increasing during inspiration, and diminishing in expiration. More interestingly, this activity can be shown to *precede* by a few milliseconds, the activation of the diaphragm (i.e. it occurs before airflow begins and before any local negative pressure sensors could be responsible for activating it), as if pre-activating the upper airway muscles in preparation for the impending negative pressure of inspiration. It is now thought that the pharyngeal dilators, in addition to the diaphragm, comprise the efferent output of the respiratory centre. Moreover, both hypoxic and hypercapnic drive to the respiratory centre, via stimulation of central and carotid body chemoreceptors, produce just as much increase in phasic efferent drive to the pharyngeal dilators as they do to the diaphragm. It is now clear that both *central* control of ventilation and control of airway patency are intimately linked.

The effect of central depressant drugs

It is well known that anaesthetic agents and opiates depress minute ventilation and the hypoxic ventilatory response via actions on the afferent sensor (peripheral chemoreceptor) and the central processor (respiratory centre). The net effect is a diminished efferent output of the phrenic nerve. However, there is also evidence that which ever drugs suppress ventilatory drive also suppress in parallel the efferent output to the pharyngeal dilators to various degrees. There is no consistent pattern as to which of these two systems is depressed most. This variability reflects the complex nature of opiate actions on the control of breathing. It may therefore be over-simplistic to categorize sleep/anaesthetic apnoeas

as either 'central' or 'obstructive', since the latter may just be the expression of the former.

Key points

- Flow tends to be turbulent in upper airway obstruction, so gas density is influential.
- The human upper airway has a 'collapsible' segment – the pharynx.
- Maintenance of pharyngeal airway patency is a complex neuromuscular phenomenon.
- Expiratory flow is less affected than inspiratory flow in upper airway obstruction; venting of gases through the upper airway is rarely a problem during trans-tracheal jet ventilation.
- In airway obstruction at pharyngeal level, inspiratory flow may not be increased by increased inspiratory effort, but can be increased by positive pressure applied above the obstruction.

Further reading

Bartlett Jr D, St John WM. Influence of morphine on respiratory activities of phrenic and hypoglossal nerves in cats. *Respir Physiol* 1986; **64**: 289–294.

Eastwood PR, Szollosi I, Platt PR, Hillman DR. Collapsibility of the upper airway during anesthesia with isoflurane. *Anesthesiology* 2002; **97**: 786–793.

Fogel R, Malhotra A, Shea S, Edwards J, White D. Reduced genioglossal activity with upper airway anesthesia in awake patients with OSA. *J Appl Physiol* 2000; **88**: 1346–1354.

Ho MH, Lee A, Karmakar MK *et al.* Heliox vs air-oxygen mixtures for the treatment of patients with acute asthma. *Chest* 2003; **123**: 882–890.

Malhotra A, Fogel R, Edwards J, Shea S, White D. Local mechanisms drive genioglossus activation in obstructive sleep apnea. *Am J Respir Crit Care Med.* 2000; **161**: 1746–1749.

Mathru M, Esch O, Lang J *et al.* Magnetic resonance imaging of the upper airway. Effects of propofol anesthesia and nasal continuous positive airway pressure in humans. *Anesthesiology* 1996; **84**: 273–279.

Nandi PR, Charlesworth CH, Taylor SJ, Nunn JF, Dore CJ. Effect of general anaesthesia on the pharynx. *Br J Anaesth* 1991; **66**: 157–162.

A. Pearce

Decontamination is the combination of processes, including cleaning, disinfection and/or sterilization, used to render a reusable medical device safe for further use. It is important because of the risk of transmission of hospital acquired infections and transmissible spongiform encephalopathies. The recommendations of the Department of Health are clear and detail that single use disposable airway equipment should be used where possible. Where this is not possible, equipment should be sterilized by heat (autoclave) and where this is not possible cold, chemical sterilization or disinfection by an automated process should be used. The term disinfection means the elimination of all vegetative pathogenic organisms such as bacteria and viruses, and sterilization indicates the elimination of all pathogens including spores. For a terminally sterilized medical device to be labelled sterile, the theoretical probability of there being a viable microorganism present on the device should be equal to or less than 1×10^{-6}.

An additional infective agent, the abnormal prion protein PrP^{Sc}, has great public health implications as it is the probable mechanism of transmission of variant Creutzfeldt–Jakob disease (vCJD). This prion protein cannot be eliminated by chemical means or temperatures reached in the standard autoclave. Temperatures approaching those required for incineration are needed. Reusable equipment should never be used in patients known or suspected of having vCJD unless the equipment is to be destroyed after use. In the case of flexible fibrescopes, dedicated endoscopes may be obtained from the National CJD Surveillance Unit in Edinburgh. All trusts should have Infection Control Committees and Teams which are responsible for preparing infection control policies to conform to all national and international standards and recommendations.

Single use, disposable

Single use equipment eliminates the risk of cross infection between patients through the airway device. It has become standard for tracheal tubes, oral and nasopharyngeal airways, catheter mounts, breathing filters/humidifiers, plastic facemasks, bougies, airway exchange catheters and suction apparatus. It is easy to envisage that all breathing systems, laryngoscope blades, laryngeal masks and facemasks will become single use in future, and the advances here are limited by cost or supply pressures and concerns about the comparable clinical performance of single use vs. reusable airway devices (such as the bougie). Items marked for single use only may not be re-used without compromising the Trust Clinical Negligence Scheme or exposing patients to the risk of cross infection. Various disposable sheaths have been developed which fit over rigid and flexible fibrescopes, but they are not popular and tend to decrease the transmitted light intensity.

Of particular concern is the risk of transmission of vCJD between patients. The tonsillar bed has been identified as a site in which prions may reside, leading to a recommendation from the Royal College of Anaesthetists that equipment for tonsillectomy which may become blood contaminated during or at the end of the procedure, including the laryngoscope, should be disposable. A similar recommendation was applied to the surgical instruments used in tonsillectomy, but this had an unforeseen consequence. The disposable surgical equipment was not of the same standard or design as the reusable instruments and there was a rise in the incidence of post-tonsillectomy bleeding.

Single use items have additional benefits of being sterile (often by γ irradiation) and packed ready for

use, and do not require the laborious process of cleaning and sterilization. However, they present the problems of ordering, storage and disposal of large volumes of stock.

Heat sterilization

Sufficient heat will destroy viruses, bacteria and spores but may damage thermally sensitive equipment such as flexible fibrescopes. Repeated cycles of heat sterilization will produce loss of transmitted light in rigid laryngoscope bundles. It remains the mainstay for surgical equipment (too expensive for single use status) but is commonly used currently for reusable laryngeal masks (classic, Proseal and Intubating), laryngoscope blades and handles without batteries, black rubber facemasks, rubber or silicone catheter mounts and Magill forceps. While dry-heat may be used, it is more common to use saturated steam under pressure.

The process starts with instrument cleaning to remove all blood, tissue or body fluids from the instrument. Studies from surgical instruments which are ready for use have shown that many are still contaminated with blood or tissue from previous patients. This is extremely worrying when one considers that prions are not destroyed by the temperatures reached in normal autoclaving. Apparently clean reusable anaesthetic equipment such as laryngeal masks and laryngoscope blades can be contaminated with a deposit which stains red with erythrosin, the dye which indicates the presence of plaque – a proteinaceous aggregate which rapidly develops on anything placed in the mouth (Figure 4.1). Manual cleaning, external and internal, with a scrubbing brush, warm water and detergent can be very effective but is time consuming and has no quality standard – some people are more diligent scrubbers! Immersion in a enzymatic detergent with an agitated wash or ultrasonic cleaning cycle will have a better quality standard.

Porous-load sterilizers (autoclaves) use vacuum assistance to remove air from the chamber and are suitable for all airway devices including those with

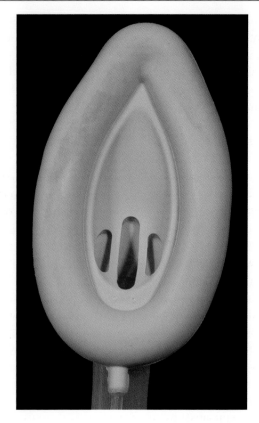

Figure 4.1 Pink staining proteinaceous material on 'clean' reusable laryngeal mask.

lumens (e.g. laryngeal masks). The stages of the operating cycle are air evacuation, sterilizing and post-vacuum or drying. A typical cycle incorporates a temperature of 134–138°C held for 12 min. Simple bench-top sterilizers without vacuum assistance are unsuitable for wrapped loads or devices with lumens. Regular functional testing of the sterilizer is required. This is aided by chemical process indicators which may be distributed within the test load and demonstrate a change of colour when exposed to heat. The chemical indicators may be autoclave tape, test tubes containing chemical indicator or sterilization bags.

Cold chemical sterilization

If devices are not single use and may not be autoclaved, cold chemical sterilization is used. Intubating fibrescopes are now the only commonly used airway equipment sterilized in this manner. Until recently the standard agent was 2% activated glutaraldehyde and, after cleaning with detergent, the fibrescope was fully immersed for 10–20 min. This immersion time was considered suitable for vegetative organisms but was ineffective against spores so that these immersion times allowed disinfection but not sterilization. Glutaraldehyde vaporizes easily and is toxic, irritant and allergenic. The Control of Substances Hazardous to Health (COSHH) Regulations 1988 limits occupational atmospheric exposure to 0.05 ppm. Developments in cold sterilizing chemicals have concentrated on killing all organisms (sterilization), reducing the stand-time to no more than 5–10 min, making the agents nontoxic to healthcare professionals, patients and to the fibrescopes themselves. Substances include peracetic acid (NuCidex, Gigasept, Perasafe), orthophthaladehyde (Cidex-OPA), super-oxidized water (Sterilox) and chlorine dioxide (Tristel).

Immediately after use the fibrescope should be decontaminated by thorough manual washing/scrubbing of the external surface and working channel in a low-foaming, enzymatic detergent solution to remove blood and mucus, because disinfectants do not penetrate mucus. Any suction valves should be removed and disassembled for cleaning and the working channel cleaned with an appropriate single use channel cleaning brush.

The scope is rinsed with water to remove the detergent and taken to an automated disinfector which generally starts with a detergent cycle and rinse (including irrigation of the working channel), followed by a stand-time of appropriate length in the disinfectant or sterilant. A final rinse with sterile or filtered water renders the fibrescope ready for reuse. Automated processes are superior to manual cleaning because they are more open to quality control. A label indicating satisfactory cleaning should be attached to the patient's notes along with a record of the fibrescope identity, and a patient register should be maintained for each fibrescope. This allows tracking of the clinical use of a fibrescope. Irrigation of the working channel with isopropyl

alcohol is recommended before the scope is stored in a dry environment, without the suction valve in place and with the insertion tube hanging down to let the working channel dry out. Fibrescopes are stored in non-sterile cupboards and it is recommended that if the interval between disinfection and elective clinical use is more than a few hours, the fibrescope should undergo another automated sterilization cycle before use.

Ethylene oxide

Ethylene oxide is a flammable, colourless gas at temperatures above 11°C. It possesses good sterilant properties but has a number of serious disadvantages. The gas is flammable and toxic causing eye pain, sore throat, dizziness, nausea, headache, convulsions and death in high concentrations. It is also carcinogenic. It may be used for thermally sensitive equipment such as an intubating fibrescope. However, the cycle time for gassing and degassing is several days and stock levels must take account of this.

Key points

- Cross infection may occur through reusable airway devices.
- Airway equipment should be single use disposable when possible.
- Reusable equipment should be heat sterilized if possible.
- Porous-load autoclaves are required for equipment with lumens.
- Chemical disinfection is required for fibrescopes.
- Automated disinfectors should be used for fibrescopes.
- Abnormal prion proteins are not destroyed by standard autoclave or chemical disinfection cycles.

Further reading

Blunt MC, Burchett KR. Variant Creutzfeldt–Jakob disease and disposable anaesthetic equipment – balancing the risks. *Br J Anaesth* 2003; **90**: 1–3.

British Society of Gastroenterology guidelines for decontamination of equipment for gastrointestinal endoscopy (2003): available on www.bsg.org.uk

Bucx MJ, Dankert J, Beenhakker MM, Harrison TE. Decontamination of laryngoscopes in the Netherlands. *Br J Anaesth* 2001; **86**: 99–102.

Miller DM, Youkhana I, Karunaratne WU, Pearce A. Presence of protein deposits on 'cleaned' reusable anaesthetic equipment. *Anaesthesia* 2001; **56**: 1069–1072.

I. Calder & A. Pearce

There are as many opinions as there are people: each has his own correct way

Terence ca. 190–159 BC

That may be right in theory, but it will not work in practice

From an essay title by Immanuel Kant 1793

Serious problems with airway management are rare, but situations that have the potential to have a bad outcome are not uncommon. Most anaesthetists are exposed to a 'just barely in control' airway situation from time to time, and there is an element of becoming 'sadder and wiser' in many anaesthetic careers. Anaesthetists are increasingly exposed to legal action in the event of an unfavourable outcome. They are therefore inclined to adopt procedures that will be supported by a substantial majority of their peers, however because of the infrequency of serious airway problems it is difficult to compare one technique with another in a rigorous way and be certain of a 'best buy'. Most techniques work in most situations. All will fail sometimes. We have no solid 'evidence base' to guide us. For instance, accepted canons of management such as the 'rapid sequence induction' (RSI) with cricoid pressure have never been subjected to a trial.

Most techniques require training and practice. It is hard both to obtain and provide training – and getting harder. Ethical constraints loom larger and larger and the trainee's time is increasingly at a premium. The advent of the laryngeal mask airway (LMA) has revolutionized anaesthesia, but it cannot be denied that most of us get less practice in mask anaesthesia and tracheal intubation than before its introduction.

There are some tenets that are based on accumulated experience.

1 *Preparation is paramount*: this includes ensuring that the correct staff are available as well as equipment.
2 *Pre-oxygenation gives valuable extra time for establishment of a patent airway.*
3 *Good monitoring equipment almost certainly reduces the frequency of serious complications.*
4 *The airway should be expected to become less patent when the conscious level declines*: this is almost always the case, with the occasional exception of patients who are panicking. However, the vast majority are easy to control with simple measures.
5 *In general there are fewer problems with the airway when patients are deeply anaesthetized.* An analogy with safety in a submarine is often drawn.
6 *Aspiration of material into the lungs becomes a possibility when the conscious level declines*: separation of the airway from the pharynx becomes more worthwhile as the risk increases.
7 *If difficulty with an airway is possible, consideration should be given to regional or local anaesthesia.*
8 *If the airway is likely to be uncontrollable with face mask, supra-glottic device or direct laryngoscopic introduction of a tracheal tube after induction, then a tracheal airway should be established before induction*: the problem here is the definition of 'likely'. Those skilled in blind techniques may disagree.

Approaches to airway management

There is a spectrum of airway management. At one end is the establishment of femoro–femoro cardiopulmonary bypass (CPB) before induction. Then there is 'awake' placement of a tracheal tube or tracheostomy. After that there is maintenance of spontaneous breathing by inducing with inhalational agents. Following that there is intravenous induction but eschewing muscle-relaxant drugs, lest the patient prove difficult to ventilate. At the other end is the concept of taking charge of the airway and imposing one's will on the situation by immediate abolition of airway reflexes. The classic RSI, where induction is intravenous and muscle paralysis is profound, is the obvious example.

An ideal technique would allow retreat at any time if success is not achieved, but experience suggests that half-hearted interventions are to be condemned, so that it is often difficult to satisfy both the desire to keep the procedure reversible and the necessity of achieving a safe level of anaesthesia.

CPB

Femoro–femoro CPB can be instituted under local anaesthesia to allow oxygenation while an airway is obtained. This technique has been used with acute airway obstruction due to massive goitres and tracheal trauma.

'Awake' intubation

Commonly performed with a flexible fibreoptic laryngoscope. Tracheostomy under local, or retrograde intubation are alternatives when a view cannot be obtained with a 'scope'.

'Awake' intubation and the obstructed airway: There are at least three reasons why awake intubation may not be the best choice. Firstly, topical application of lidocaine to the airway does sometimes make the quality of the airway worse. Secondly, approaching a glottis with a 'scope can provoke obstruction, especially if topicalization has been inadequate. However, there will always be exceptions – a patient with ankylosing spondylitis and epiglottitis, for instance. Rigid bronchoscopy under local anaesthesia may be the best choice when central mediastinal masses are causing obstruction. Thirdly, if a patient with borderline airway patency begins to panic the situation becomes worse, so awake procedures may not be tolerated.

Induction with inhalational agents

The prospect of finding oneself unable to ventilate an apnoeic patient concentrates the mind. So the idea of preserving spontaneous breathing until it is possible to show that either tracheal intubation can be performed, or that one can ventilate with a mask or LMA, is a sensible one. However, it is a common finding that patients can be ventilated with positive pressure when it is very difficult to maintain an airway with spontaneous ventilation, because the increased negative inspiratory intra-thoracic pressure collapses the airway (see Chapter 3). The phenomenon of obstructive sleep apnoea being relieved by continuous airway positive pressure (CPAP) is an example. Nevertheless, many practitioners with experience of obstructed airways recommend a spontaneously breathing technique.

There are many who believe that propofol is such an airway-friendly drug, that careful intravenous administration is preferable for trying to achieve a safe depth of anaesthesia via an already impaired airway. Hari and Nirvala reported a case of retropharyngeal abscess, in which the airway became completely obstructed during inhalational induction, but was relieved by intravenous propofol. It is widely accepted that intravenous propofol is an excellent treatment for airway obstruction due to laryngospasm.

Glottic closure reflexes must be obtunded before instrumentation and the margin between adequate glottic anaesthesia and apnoea in a spontaneously breathing patient is small. It is probable that we cannot avoid the possibility of rendering a patient apnoeic whether we use an inhalational or an intravenous technique.

Intravenous induction/muscle paralysis

A career in anaesthesia without access to muscle-relaxant drugs would be unattractive to most. In the vast majority of cases of difficulty with the airway, muscle relaxants are not the problem; in fact, they are the solution. The ability to suppress airway reflexes promptly and enable positive pressure ventilation to be easily performed is a very valuable feature of these drugs, indeed in many hospitals it is policy to have succinylcholine drawn up ready at all times. In the standard RSI the ability to ventilate with a mask is not determined before administration of a muscle relaxant. Succinylcholine is still used for this purpose, on the grounds that its action begins and terminates more quickly than with non-depolarizing agents. Whether the action of succinylcholine reliably terminates quickly enough to prevent hypoxic damage is debated, but the chances are better than with the non-depolarizers. It has been suggested that the dose generally used ($1\,mg\,kg^{-1}$) could be reduced to $0.56\,mg\,kg^{-1}$, allowing even more rapid termination, without making intubation more difficult.

Despite their overall benefit, the worry with muscle relaxants is that both ventilation and tracheal intubation will prove impossible. There are some patients who are so obviously likely to be difficult to ventilate that it would be foolish to give muscle relaxants, unless all other avenues had been exhausted. There is no 'never' in medicine – for instance the case of Ludwig's angina described by Neff *et al.* where the airway obstruction consequent on the abscess bursting during induction was relieved by succinylcholine.

Patients who do not look obviously abnormal, but are impossible to ventilate, are extremely rare. Some practitioners find that they can manage without muscle relaxants, since the combination of propofol and powerful opioids allows tracheal intubation. Adnet *et al.* used midazolam $0.03\,mg\,kg^{-1}$, sufentanyl $0.25\,\mu g\,kg^{-1}$ and propofol $2.5\,mg\,kg^{-1}$ to successfully intubate 456 patients. However, the rate of difficult laryngoscopy was 11%, which is high, and suggests that one risk is being exchanged for another.

Establishing that ventilation is possible before giving muscle relaxants: it is comforting to know that mask ventilation will be possible before giving a muscle relaxant, and this has become a common practice. It will not be possible to prove that this tactic is effective in reducing episodes of impossible ventilation because of the small number of true cases. A counter argument is that the practice will result in an increase in poorly controlled airways, since muscle relaxants are the most effective way of abolishing unwanted reflexes such as breath holding and the stiffness associated with opioids. Nevertheless, anecdotal evidence supports the practice. A consultant anaesthetist was disciplined after a fatal outcome when he gave a patient, who was expected to have a difficult airway, a large dose of a non-depolarizing agent, and found that he could not ventilate or intubate the patient. However, it is unwise to be too dogmatic about these issues, since we may jeopardize patients by training anaesthetists to be scared of giving muscle relaxants. In the authors' experience difficulty with an airway is most often due to *inadequate* doses of agents, including muscle relaxants.

Planning airway management

The steps envisaged as leading to safe management of the airway were postulated by the American Society of Anesthesiologists (ASA) in 1993. Over the last 10 years extensive critical thought has gone into the validation or rejection of the way of thinking proposed by this document and there is much to reject. What has remained valid is the idea that good management of the airway requires the anaesthetist to consider a number of steps or phases.

Steps in airway management (ASA)

- Evaluation of the airway.
- Preparation for difficulty.
- Airway strategy at the start of 'anaesthesia'.
- Airway strategy at the end of 'anaesthesia'.
- Follow-up.

Evaluation of the patient seeks to establish which airway device will provide the appropriate level of airway protection and maintenance for the proposed surgery, and whether there will be any difficulty. In most cases, excluding shared airway scenarios, the airway is always managed by either face mask, supraglottic airway such as the LMA or tracheal intubation. A tracheal tube generally gives the highest level of airway protection and maintenance, and for this reason figures highly in resuscitation and anaesthetic practice. It also figures highly in deaths related to airway management. It has been suggested (by the manufacturers) that 200 million laryngeal masks have been inserted without any death directly attributed to insertion of the mask. It is impossible to make such a claim for tracheal intubation.

The decision as to which airway device is appropriate for the planned surgery is made through experience but is determined by the size of the patient and the perceived risk of aspiration, the nature of surgery and whether positive pressure ventilation is required, the requirement for surgical access around the head or neck, whether surgery is likely to interfere with the airway, personal preference or experience and factors such as 'are you feeling lucky?'. There are substantial variations between anaesthetists as to their view of the correct way to manage the airway. A specimen scenario might be that of a 100 kg patient undergoing diagnostic laparoscopy – can the airway be managed safely by laryngeal mask or is tracheal intubation required?

Evaluation of the airway to predict difficulty is covered in detail in Chapter 15 but it is important to realize that evaluation of the patient is the only factor which will determine what strategy an individual anaesthetist (working in a particular environment) will adopt. Predicting difficulty may lead to postponement of surgery, undertaking surgery under local or regional anaesthesia, assembling additional help or equipment, planning ways of managing the airway and allows discussion with the patient about possible options. Evaluation is an imperfect process so that patients regarded as normal may not be, and patients predicted to be difficult may not be. It is airway strategy which copes with the unreliability of evaluation and our plans must cope with unanticipated difficulty and any plans used in cases of difficulty must not damage 'normal' patients.

Airway strategy

Strategy indicates a combination of plans (Plans A and B) which, together, should lead to a live patient without morbidity. The times of particular problem are at the initiation and termination of general anaesthesia and there should be specific strategies at these two stages. Most patients are regarded as normal on pre-operative evaluation and the anaesthetist

selects their 'default' strategy – that which they do when no difficulty is anticipated. If face mask anaesthesia is Plan A and this proves unsatisfactory, Plan B is often to insert a laryngeal mask. If Plan A is insertion of a laryngeal mask and this proves to be unsatisfactory, Plan B is usually tracheal intubation. If tracheal intubation is required in Plan A and this fails, it is possible to make a decision that the operation can, after all, be undertaken with a laryngeal mask. Generally, however, if tracheal intubation is considered to be the correct level of airway maintenance and protection it may be considered desirable for Plan B also. Part of the 'uniqueness' of tracheal intubation is that there are many techniques for placing a tube in the trachea and if one fails we can move to another. Unfortunately, familiarity with techniques of intubation other than by direct laryngoscopy is not widespread. Managing the airway at the end of anaesthesia is considered in Chapter 10.

Algorithms and flowcharts

One of the ways of producing some structure to the way in which we think about managing normal and difficult airways is by algorithm or flowchart. A version of the ASA algorithm is shown in Figure 5.1. It can be seen that difficult airway management may be anticipated or unanticipated. If *anticipated* the airway should be managed in a certain way and if *unanticipated*, differentiation should be made between difficult ventilation and difficult intubation because the management of these two situations is quite different.

There are several problems with difficult airway guidelines and algorithms. There is the initial problem of what is meant by a normal or difficult airway. A difficult airway generally incorporates either difficult face mask ventilation or difficult intubation (or both) and common definitions or meanings of these are given in Chapter 15. Difficult intubation is virtually always taken as difficult direct laryngoscopy, but there may be sub-glottic causes of difficult intubation or intubation may be easy by another technique. To label someone as a 'difficult intubation' when it can be accomplished within 20 s with an intubating LMA (ILMA) is bizarre. The term difficult direct laryngoscopy at least narrows the problem down to

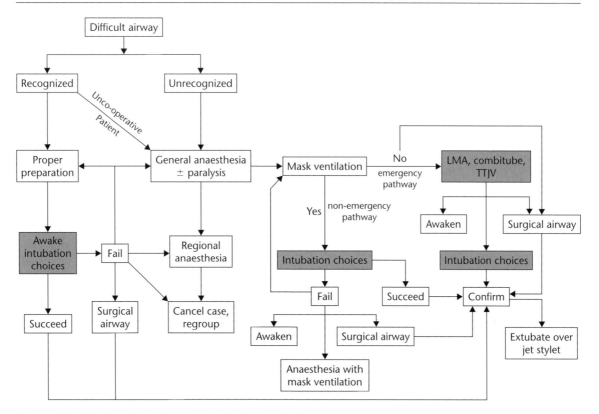

Figure 5.1 ASA algorithm. TTJV: transtracheal jet ventilation.

not having a clear view of the larynx by direct view with a Macintosh or straight-blade laryngoscope.

While flowcharts are very fashionable, it has not been shown that they actually improve airway management. They are of course well intentioned, but sometimes represent a wish-list of expertise or equipment. Difficult airway algorithms often include techniques such as 'fibreoptic intubation' or 'use the Bullard', and if the reader does not possess this particular skill, the algorithm is without value.

In order to be useful, it is probable that difficult airway flowcharts should use only a range of core skills which are in the training syllabus, that the flowchart addresses a well-defined common airway scenario and that the chart contains information about the individual steps. Flowcharts, appropriate to the UK, describing routine or default intubation strategy, failed RSI and failed ventilation have been produced recently by the Difficult Airway Society

(DAS) and are available as a published article and also on the DAS web site (www.das.uk.com).

Routine or default intubation strategy

One of the DAS flowcharts covers the commonest clinical scenario which gives rise to problems, that of routine intubation in an elective surgical patient not anticipated to be difficult to manage (Figure 5.2). The flowchart is applicable, therefore, to most patients undergoing tracheal intubation in an operating theatre environment. In Plan A of this situation oxygenation is supplied by face mask ventilation around intubation attempts, intubation is attempted by optimal direct laryngoscopy, laryngeal reflexes are abolished by muscle relaxation and patient distress overcome by general anaesthesia. If face mask ventilation proves impossible after the induction of general anaesthesia with muscle relaxation, Plan B for failed ventilation is activated – an ascending sequence

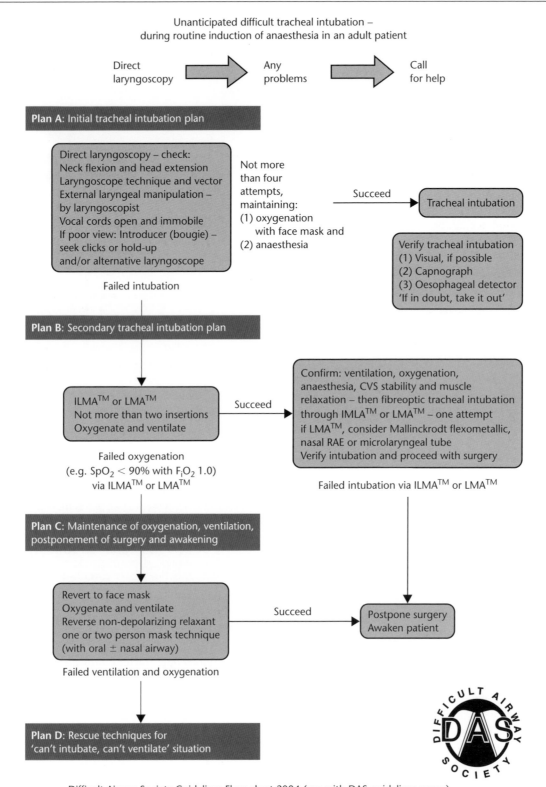

Difficult Airway Society Guidelines Flow-chart 2004 (use with DAS guidelines paper)

Figure 5.2 DAS flowchart. CVS: cardiovascular system.

of oral airway, two- to four-handed face mask ventilation, laryngeal mask insertion and emergency cricothyrotomy. If intubation fails by optimal direct laryngoscopy, Plan B starts by placing a laryngeal mask (classic or intubating) and ensuring oxygenation, anaesthesia, muscle relaxation and appropriate control of cardiovascular parameters and arterial CO_2 before proceeding to use that airway as a route for intubation. If it is not possible to place an LMA or ILMA, or not possible to intubate through it, the patient is awoken and the surgery rescheduled.

In selecting techniques for inclusion into flowcharts, a number of common-sense decisions can be made. The prevalence of failure to intubate by direct laryngoscopy aided by a bougie, in a trained anaesthetist, is probably only about $1:500$–2000 in general surgical patients in whom no problem is predicted. This means that an 'average' anaesthetist will fail to intubate in a general surgical patient no more commonly than once every 3–5 years. It is preferable for any intubation technique to be visual rather than blind, to allow easy ventilation around or during attempts at intubation, for mannikin practice of the technique to be useful in training for clinical use, to use equipment present in every hospital and to enable as many transferable skills as possible such that the core repertoire of an anaesthetist is kept to a small number of complementary techniques. Possibly the best manager of the airway is the person who has the fewest number of well-practised strategies to cover the largest number of clinical scenarios.

Follow-up

Documentation of the airway component of anaesthetic care will include a pre-operative airway evaluation, checking of the breathing system, anaesthetic machine and suction, auxiliary ventilating bag and setting of relevant monitors. The ease of face mask inflation, laryngeal mask insertion or intubation should be noted. It is usual to record the Cormack and Lehane grade of laryngeal view.

When difficulty with airway management has been encountered, more detailed notes and follow-up

should be initiated. The anaesthetic records should detail the problem encountered and how it was solved, noting specifically whether face mask ventilation was possible under anaesthesia. A note should be made contemporaneously in the hospital records. The patient needs to be reviewed so that any morbidity can be found and treated, with an explanation to the patient of what problem was encountered. The patient should be encouraged to remember that difficulty was encountered and to tell the next anaesthetist. A letter to the patient, copied to the general practitioner, hospital notes and to a department register should repeat the oral explanation. If the problem is serious or life threatening, will recur with future anaesthetics and is not obvious from external examination the patient should be encouraged to join Medic Alert and wear a bracelet inscribed with 'difficult intubation' or 'difficult airway'. It is easiest to use a form for this and one is available on the DAS web site (www.das.uk.com) used with permission from the authors who described the form in 2003.

Key points

- Planning ahead is vital.
- Assemble the correct equipment and staff.
- Be flexible.
- Utilize any training opportunity.

Further reading

Adnet F, Baillard C, Borron SW et al. Randomized study comparing the 'sniffing position' with simple head extension for laryngoscopic view in elective surgery patients. Anesthesiology 2001; 95: 836–841.

Belmont MJ, Wax MK, DeSouza FN. The difficult airway: cardiopulmonary bypass – the ultimate solution. Head Neck 1998; 20: 266–269.

Benumof JL. Preoxygenation: best method for both efficacy and efficiency. Anesthesiology 1999; 91: 603–605.

Benumof JL, Dagg R, Benumof R. Critical hemoglobin desaturation will occur before return to an unparalyzed state following 1 mg/kg intravenous succinylcholine. Anesthesiology 1997; 87: 979–982.

Conacher ID, Curran E. Local anaesthesia and sedation for rigid bronchoscopy for emergency relief of central airway obstruction. *Anaesthesia* 2004; **59**: 290–292.

Donati F. The right dose of succinylcholine. *Anesthesiology* 2003; **99**: 1037–1038.

Goodwin MW, Pandit JJ, Hames K, Popat M, Yentis SM. The effect of neuromuscular blockade on the efficiency of manual ventilation of the lungs. *Anaesthesia* 2003; **58**: 60–63.

Gurung AM, Tomlinson AA. Pre-preparation of succinylcholine: significant waste for questionable benefit. *Anaesthesia* 2004; **59**: 211–212.

Hari MS, Nirvala KD. Retropharyngeal abscess presenting with acute airway obstruction. *Anaesthesia* 2003; **58**: 712–713.

Mason RA, Fielden CP. The obstructed airway in head and neck surgery. *Anaesthesia* 54: 625–628.

Neff SPW, Merry AF, Anderson B. Airway management in Ludwig's angina. *Anaesth Intens Care* 1999; **27**: 659–661.

Ricard-Hibon A, Chollet C, Leroy C, Marty J. Succinylcholine improves the time of performance of a tracheal intubation in prehospital critical care medicine. *Eur J Anaesthesiol* 2002; **19**: 361–367.

Stringer KR, Bajenov S, Yentis SM. Training in airway management. *Anaesthesia* 2002; **57**: 1967–1983.

T.M. Cook

Effect of induction on the airway

The induction of general anaesthesia or sedation tends to result in hypoxia because of:

1 Airway obstruction. Maintenance of a patent upper airway is a complex physiological mechanism. Even minor depression of consciousness can result in obstruction.
2 Respiratory depression.
3 Decreased cardiac output.

Mechanism of airway obstruction

It is a usual practice to induce anaesthesia with the patient supine and nearly horizontal, which is the least favourable position for airway patency, but the most convenient for intervention. Relaxation of the musculature of the pharynx, face and neck allows the soft palate, tongue and glottic opening to approach the posterior nasopharyngeal wall. The greatest contribution to obstruction is believed to be at glottic and velo–palatine level.

Signs of airway obstruction

1 An obstructed upper airway results in increases in negative intrathoracic pressure during inspiration. This causes tracheal 'tug', intercostal and supra-clavicular recession and paradoxical or 'seesaw' breathing (if the airway is obstructed the chest sinks in and the abdomen rises – the opposite of normal).
2 Turbulent flow may occur in the upper airway, resulting in noise. The noise is worse on inspiration. The characteristic timbre of snoring (palatal, tongue and peri–glottic level obstruction) and stridor (glottic and tracheal level) are readily recognized with experience. Absence of noise does not mean that the airway is not critically narrowed and a completely obstructed airway is silent. Auscultation of the neck to assess airway patency is a valuable examination.
3 Secretions or foreign bodies in the airway may cause obstruction. The noise of secretions is characteristic. Foreign bodies in anaesthetic circuits (introduced by accident or malicious design) have resulted in tragedies. If airway obstruction occurs, the anaesthetist must ensure that the circuit and any artificial airway is patent.
4 It is important to realize that normal values of pulse oximetry or PaO_2 are not reliable indicators of airway patency. Tragedies have occurred when the significance of near-normal saturation in patients receiving added oxygen has not been appreciated.
5 With experience, anaesthetists can generally assess the patency of the airway by observation of the movements of the reservoir bag and the 'feel' of the bag when positive pressure is applied.

Basic airway manoeuvres

Patient positioning

As previously mentioned, the supine position is generally the best compromise between ease of intervention and airway deterioration. However, patients with respiratory insufficiency, gross obesity, or airway obstruction may find the supine position intolerable. The lateral position is preferred in advanced pregnancy to avoid the supine hypotensive syndrome.

Head extension and chin lift

Extension of the cranio-cervical junction tensions the soft tissues of the neck, which results in elevation of the glottis and peri-glottic tissues from the posterior pharyngeal wall. During chin lift a finger is placed behind the point of the chin and the bony jaw lifted anteriorly. In reality the two procedures usually occur together. A degree of flexion of the lower cervical spine, produced by placing the head on a pillow, is often helpful. This position is known as the 'sniffing position' or 'draining a pint of beer' position. The 'triple manoeuvre' describes the three elements of upper cervical extension, lower cervical flexion and jaw protrusion.

Jaw thrust

Protrusion of the mandible so that the lower incisors lie anterior to the upper incisors produces elevation of tongue, soft palate and glottis. Joseph Clover was probably the first to describe the technique in 1868. Esmarch's illustration in his *1877 Handbook of War Surgery* remains one of the best. The jaw may also be advanced by placing the thumb inside the mouth behind the lower incisors and pulling anteriorly (Figure 6.1).

During all airway clearing manoeuvres care should be taken to apply forces to bony tissues rather than soft tissues as the latter may worsen airway obstruction.

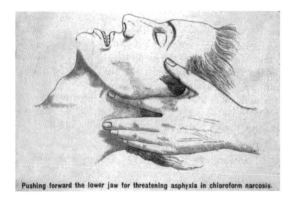

Pushing forward the lower jaw for threatening asphyxia in chloroform narcosis.

Figure 6.1 Jaw thrust. (From Esmarch F 1877. By kind permission of The Royal Society of Medicine.)

Supra-glottic airway devices

Bag and mask

The most important adjunct to airway management during anaesthesia is the bag and mask. Standard face masks are plastic or rubber cones designed to fit over the nose and mouth. A 22 mm connector allows attachment to an anaesthetic breathing circuit and an air-filled edge allows a gas-tight seal to be made with the face. Sizes range to fit infant to large adult. Most are now made of clear plastic, which affords patient comfort and allows patient colour and secretions to be observed. Specialized small masks are available that encircle only the nose and these have traditionally been popular for chair dental anaesthesia. In paediatric practice the dead-space of conventional mask becomes significant and masks such as the Baker-Rendell-Soucek mask are designed to overcome this problem.

In most cases the anaesthetist can apply the mask and control the airway with one hand. In difficult patients the anaesthetist may require both hands to control the situation.

Guedel airway

This was first described in 1933 and is a hollow partially flattened plastic tube formed in the shape of the superior surface of the tongue. It acts both to open the mouth and to lift the tongue and glottis from the hypopharynx. There are seven sizes from neonatal to large adult. Size is approximated by measuring from the midline of the mouth to the angle of the jaw. The airway is inserted upside-down (convexity downwards) in adults, until the soft palate is reached and it is then rotated 180°. This technique minimizes the risk of inadvertently forcing the tongue backwards during insertion. In children, placement under direct vision, using a tongue depressor or laryngoscope blade is preferred and this is equally suitable for adults. Insertion of a Guedel of the wrong size or in light planes of anaesthesia may lead to airway obstruction, laryngospasm or regurgitation. Damage to diseased or crowned incisor teeth can result from patients biting the airway during emergence (although this is true of all oral airway devices). The Guedel airway is designed for single use and costs <£0.50.

Nasal airway

A nasal airway is less commonly used to assist airway clearance during anaesthesia. The nasal airway should not cause blanching of the nostril when inserted and a size >7.0 mm is never necessary. The length of the airway may be estimated from the tip of the nose to tragus of the ear or 3 cm longer than an oral airway. The airway is inserted into the nostril then advanced parallel to the roof of the mouth, below the inferior turbinate. Insertion is stimulating, but once inserted a nasal airway is well tolerated and may be left in place until the patient is fully awake. The principal complication of the use of a nasal airway is bleeding, which may be profuse. Nasal airways should not be used in the presence of base of skull fractures or severe bleeding diatheses. They are designed for single use and cost £2–3.

The laryngeal mask airway and other devices

Prior to 1988 almost all general anaesthesia was conducted with face mask or tracheal tube. The classic laryngeal mask airway (cLMA) was introduced in 1988 and rapidly transformed the way in which anaesthesia is practised throughout the world. Since that time, and particularly in the last 5 years there has been an explosion of new supraglottic airway devices (SADs) designed to compete with the cLMA. These devices vary considerably in the degree to which they have been evaluated before and since marketing. Most of the devices have been modified several times since introduction, so literature on device performance must be interpreted with great care, to ensure the evaluated device is currently produced.

The majority of SADs are designed to lie with their tip at the origin of the oesophagus with the aim of 'plugging' the oesophagus. A seal around the larynx is then achieved by a more proximal cuff, which acts to elevate the base of the tongue, lift the epiglottis and seal the oropharynx. All airways that are inserted beyond the epiglottis may lead to down folding of the epiglottis and airway obstruction. One of the design challenges of these devices is to allow positioning of the distal portion of the device behind the cricoid cartilage without displacing the epiglottis during placement.

cLMA

The cLMA was designed by Dr Archie Brain in the UK in the early 1980s and introduced to anaesthetic practice in 1988. Today, having been used in approximately 150 million anaesthetics globally, the cLMA is currently the gold standard for SADs. The cLMA is made of silicone and can be used in patients with latex allergy. The cLMA is designed for use up to 40 times.

There are eight sizes of cLMA (1, 1.5, 2, 2.5, 3, 4, 5 and 6) for use from neonates to large adults. Size selection is according to patient weight (Table 6.1). Using a larger size cLMA for a given patient is likely to result in an improved laryngeal seal. Over recent years the size of mask recommended has been increased and the largest size (#6) introduced.

Dr Archie Brain (1942–)

Archie was born in Japan where his parents were diplomats. He took a degree in modern languages at Oxford before taking up medicine. He devised the LMA and ensured it entered production, despite enormous practical difficulties. He continues to work on airway devices. Archie was awarded the Magill Gold Medal of the Association of Anaesthetists in 1995 and elected as an Honorary Member in 2000.

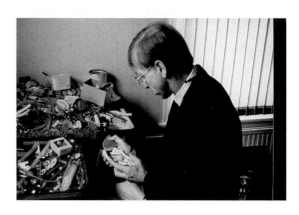

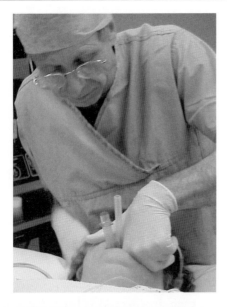

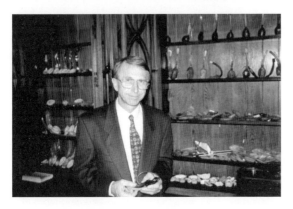

The cLMA is an alternative both to anaesthesia with face mask or tracheal tube. It is primarily designed for use during spontaneous ventilation, but it is also widely used for controlled ventilation.

The cLMA is not suitable for all cases and good case selection is the key to successful use. Most critically the cLMA should not be regarded as providing any protection against aspiration of regurgitated gastric contents and is contraindicated for patients who are not starved or who may have a full stomach. Relative contraindications include obesity, pharyngolaryngeal pathology and reduced lung compliance.

Insertion is performed with the patient in the 'sniffing position'. The cLMA should be visually inspected, and free from foreign bodies and the posterior surface lubricated. Full deflation before insertion allows the cLMA to slide behind the cricoid cartilage and reduces the likelihood of the leading edge hitting the epiglottis during insertion. The airway is held like a pen, with the index finger placed at the anterior junction of the airway tube and mask. The cLMA is inserted into the mouth and its posterior aspect pressed onto the hard palate. The index finger is then advanced towards the occiput, which causes the cLMA to pass along the roof of the mouth and then the posterior pharynx. The device is advanced in a single smooth movement until it is felt to stop, on reaching the cricopharyngeus muscle. During insertion the non-intubating hand is used to prevent flexion of the head. Chin lift or jaw thrust applied by an assistant may ease insertion. Once fully inserted the tube should be held while the intubating finger is withdrawn.

The depth of anaesthesia required for cLMA insertion is greater than that needed for insertion of a Guedel airway. Prior to insertion there should

Table 6.1 cLMA data				
Size	Patient weight	Length	*Maximum cuff volume*	Largest tracheal tube that can be passed
1	Neonate <5 kg	8	4	3.5
1.5	Infant 5–10 kg	10	7	4.0
2	Child 10–20 kg	11	10	4.5
2.5	Child 20–30 kg	12.5	14	5.0
3	Child/small adult	16	20	6.0
4	Adult 50–70 kg	16	30	6.0
5	Adult 70–100 kg	16	40	7.0
6	Adult >100 kg	16	50	7.0

be no eyelash reflex and no response to jaw thrust. Propofol is the ideal anaesthetic induction agent for insertion as it profoundly reduces airway reflexes. Addition of an opioid or intravenous lidocaine reduces the dose of induction agent needed and improves insertion conditions. Neuromuscular blocking drugs are not needed. The cLMA may also be inserted with topical anaesthesia of the airway or bilateral supra-glottic nerve blocks. Insertion (and removal) causes minimal haemodynamic response.

The cuff should be inflated before attaching the anaesthetic circuit. When correctly inserted the black line on the posterior of the cLMA will remain in the midline. During cuff inflation the device rises out of the mouth 1–3 cm and the anterior neck fills. Most of the airway seal is achieved with the first 10 ml of air inserted into the cuff. Nitrous oxide diffuses into the cuff and leads to increases in volume and pressure, particularly in the first hour of anaesthesia. High intracuff pressures for long periods may cause pharyngeal and laryngeal mucosal or nerve damage. Injuries to the lingual, hypoglossal and recurrent laryngeal nerves have been reported. These are minimized by meticulous insertion and maintenance of intracuff pressure <70 cmH$_2$O.

Once inserted ease of manual ventilation should be assessed; there should be adequate ventilation without audible gas leak. Airway pressure >20 cmH$_2$O should be avoided. Airway noise or poor filling of the reservoir bag (impaired expiration) may indicate poor placement.

Use of a bite block (rolled gauze) placed between the molar teeth is recommended until the LMA is removed. The cLMA should be secured by tape or tie to reduce the likelihood of extrusion or displacement.

Misplacement may occur due to rotation, the tip of the device bending backwards, overfolding of the epiglottis or insertion of the tip of the device into the glottis.

Careful technique reduces all these misplacements. Insertion of the tip of the device into the laryngeal inlet may mimic laryngospasm with high airway pressures, slow expiration and wheeze. The presence of the cLMA tip behind the larynx may occasionally shorten the vocal cords leading to partial extrathoracic airway obstruction during spontaneous ventilation and paradoxical cord movement during controlled ventilation. If the origin of the oesophagus lies within the bowl of the cLMA the use of controlled ventilation may lead to gastric distension. This misplacement occurs in up to 10% of cases and may not be clinically apparent.

Airway resistance with the cLMA (tube plus laryngeal resistance) is similar to that of a conventional tracheal tube. Malposition increases resistance considerably.

During emergence the cLMA is tolerated until very light planes of anaesthesia. The cLMA may be removed with the patient supine or on their side. The bite block and cLMA should be left in place until the patient regains consciousness and airway reflexes return. The cuff should be deflated as the device is removed. Airway suction is not necessary or desirable, unless secretions are excessive, as pharyngeal secretions are removed with the airway. The evidence on timing of removal of the cLMA in children is less clear and some clinicians prefer to remove the cLMA in infants and small children before emergence.

After use the cLMA should be rapidly and thoroughly cleaned before being sterilized by autoclave and stored in sterile packaging thereafter.

Insertion is successful on first attempt in >90% of cases. The LMA provides a clear airway and hands free anaesthesia in >95% of cases. In a 11,000 patient series, the cLMA was successful for airway management in 99.8% of cases. The 0.2% failure rate is lower than quoted rates of failed tracheal intubation. In the same series the incidence of airway-related critical incidents was <1 in 500 for controlled or spontaneous ventilation. The incidence of aspiration in carefully selected elective patients is variously estimated as 1 in 5–11,000, which is similar to that with tracheal tube anaesthesia (1 in 2–4000).

Movement of head and neck has little effect on the position of the cLMA over the larynx but flexion and rotation both lead to an increase in laryngeal seal pressure and intracuff pressure. Head and neck extension has the opposite effects.

Meta-analysis has been used to compare the cLMA with the tracheal tube or face mask. Advantages over the face mask include improved oxygenation and lesser hand fatigue. Advantages over tracheal intubation include improved haemodynamic stability, reduced anaesthetic requirements during maintenance, improved emergence (improved oxygenation and reduced coughing) and reduced sore throats in adults. The cLMA reduces laryngeal morbidity compared to tracheal intubation with less mechanical and neurological vocal cord dysfunction and less laryngeal discomfort. Use of a cLMA impairs mucociliary clearance less than a tracheal tube.

When first introduced the cLMA was used almost exclusively for elective patients undergoing minor peripheral surgery breathing spontaneously. The applications for cLMA use have widened greatly since then. In the UK, in 1993, 30% of all surgical cases were performed with a cLMA and in 2002 this figure had risen to 65%. In 1994 controlled ventilation was used in <50% while in some series this figure has now risen to >80%.

The use of the cLMA for controlled ventilation remains controversial. The main concern is the issue of airway protection from regurgitated gastric contents and the possibility of gastric distension during controlled ventilation with the cLMA. Detractors of the use of controlled ventilation with the cLMA point to several factors; the cLMA has been shown to modestly reduce lower oesophageal sphincter pressure; as peak airway pressure increases the risk of gastro-oesophageal insufflation increases; an early study using swallowed capsules of methylene blue as a marker reported regurgitation and soiling of the innersurface of the cLMA in 25% of patients and the cLMA bowl has a deadspace of <5 ml if regurgitation does occur. However, when oropharyngeal leak occurs during controlled ventilation with the cLMA the leak is into (and out of) the mouth in 95% of cases. Cadaver work shows the cLMA does

provide some protection from oesophageal fluid when compared to the unprotected airway. Large series have reported use of controlled ventilation in between 44% and 95% of cases with no increase in aspiration or airway-related critical incidents. Proven aspiration with the cLMA remains very infrequent. When the cLMA is used for controlled ventilation correct positioning is critical and imperfect position should not be accepted. Airway pressures should be kept to a minimum and pressures >20 cmH$_2$O avoided altogether. Since the ProSeal LMA (PLMA) became available there is a strong argument that where controlled ventilation is required this is a more suitable device than the cLMA.

Use of the cLMA for laparoscopic surgery is also controversial. The use of controlled ventilation, raised intra-abdominal pressure and the lithotomy position all contribute to this controversy. Several small trials support the use of the cLMA for gynaecological laparoscopy and suggest muscular relaxation with controlled ventilation, or spontaneous ventilation are both acceptable techniques. The safety of the technique has not been proved but series of up to 1500 cases without aspiration are reported. In 1996, 60% of UK anaesthetists routinely used the cLMA for gynaecological laparoscopy.

The breadth of cases that the cLMA has been used for is enormous. In addition to a full range of peripheral surgery there are reports of the use of the cLMA for elective laparotomy, abdominal aortic aneurysm repair, caesarean section, neurosurgery and cardiac surgery. In intensive care medicine the cLMA has been used for brief periods of controlled ventilation in selected cases, after extubation following neurosurgery, as an aid for weaning from mechanical ventilation and during percutaneous dilational tracheostomy. However successful use does not indicate safety or even efficacy.

The cLMA is also used to maintain the airway after tracheal extubation. Tracheal extubation can cause undesirable haemodynamic complications, coughing and oxygen desaturation. The cLMA may be inserted posterior to the tracheal tube (using the tracheal tube as a guide), before extubation with a reduction in these complications.

In addition to its role during the maintenance of anaesthesia the cLMA is a useful device for gaining access to the trachea and for management of difficult airways. In 75–90% of cases the larynx is visible from the bowl of the cLMA. This allows access to the trachea either with a small tracheal tube, a bougie or exchange catheter. This has led to the use of the cLMA as a conduit (dedicated airway) during blind attempts at tracheal intubation, elective fibreoptic intubation and for bronchoscopy. Techniques using a fibrescope, allowing the procedure to be performed under direct vision are preferable, as blind access is unreliable. In the emergency setting after failed intubation the cLMA may be used as a rescue device. After failed tracheal intubation the priority is oxygenation and the cLMA is usually effective in establishing the airway. The cLMA is cited as a rescue device in the algorithm for management of failed tracheal intubation in the USA, Canada and the UK. In this context several points should be noted:

1 The tip of the LMA seats behind the cricoid cartilage. Cricoid pressure therefore impedes its placement. Cricoid pressure should be reduced or removed before placing the cLMA. Once placed, cricoid pressure may be reapplied, but may interfere with effective ventilation.
2 The LMA does not reliably protect against aspiration and where this risk is high a more secure airway will be needed.
3 In patients with difficult to manage airways, controlled ventilation may be difficult with the cLMA, in particular if high airway pressures are required there may be considerable airway leak.

The cLMA costs approximately £90.

Single use cLMAs

The main driving force for the introduction of single use devices has been concern over sterility of cleaned reusable devices. This has been a particular issue in the UK since 2001 with doubts over the elimination of proteinaceous material and the risk of transmission of prion disease. There are three manufacturers of single use cLMAs and as many as 12 are expected. Designs differ slightly between manufacturers. For patent reasons, all except those made by Intavent Orthofix do not have the epiglottic bars at the distal end of the airway tube. Particularly with the larger sizes there is a possibility of entrapping the tongue and drawing it backwards during insertion as well as obstruction by the epiglottis. For cost reasons, most single use cLMAs are made with a polyvinyl chloride (PVC) cuff which increases the rigidity of the device. The device manufactured by Marshalls retains the silicone cuff. There is no robust evidence as to whether the currently available single-use devices perform similarly to equivalent reusable devices, nor which single-use device performs best.

Each device costs between £5 and £10.

The flexible (reinforced) LMA

The flexible or reinforced LMA (fLMA) is identical to the cLMA except for the airway tube, which is made of soft silicone with spiral wire reinforcement. The airway tube is more flexible and does not kink when bent.

The fLMA is available in sizes 2–5.

Insertion technique is identical to the cLMA. Insertion success, airway position and seal pressures are similar to the cLMA, but the flexible tube is prone to axial rotation during insertion. Unless care is taken the mask may face backwards. This is, surprisingly, not always evident until removal, but reduces performance and safety. A variety of aids to placement have been reported – most recently the 'flexiguide', a rigid metal introducer which inserts into all sizes of fLMA and anchors the distal ends by means of a retractable flange has been reported to improve insertion.

The fLMA is particularly suitable for intra-oral (maxillofacial and ear, nose and throat (ENT) surgery) and nasal surgery. The airway tube can be moved as necessary to improve surgical access. The cuff of the fLMA provides good protection of the larynx from pharyngeal secretions or blood. An example of this is in tonsillectomy, where tracheal soiling is reduced when using a fLMA in comparison to a tracheal tube. Head and neck movement have little effect on the position of the mask over the larynx and recovery is smoother than with a tracheal tube with less coughing, laryngospasm, airway obstruction and hypoxia. All these features make the fLMA the airway of choice for many operations on the face or within the mouth, nose or ears.

Despite these potential advantages great care must be taken when surgical access is close to the airway. Displacement of the fLMA may lead to airway leak or obstruction. In particular placing a Boyle-Davis gag for tonsillectomy may lead to loss of the airway, requiring repositioning of the gag or mask, in 5–10% of cases.

The fLMA is a suitable airway for ophthalmic surgery. In addition to providing good surgical access the fLMA causes less rise in intra-ocular pressure and is associated with less coughing and hypoxia during emergence, than when using a tracheal tube.

Like the cLMA, the fLMA is designed for 40 uses. It costs approximately £135.

The intubating LMA

The intubating LMA (ILMA) (Fastrach™) was designed by Dr Archie Brain and introduced into practice in the late 1990s. It is designed to provide a dedicated airway and allow placement of a moderate size tracheal tube, in patients with both easy and difficult airways (Figure 6.2).

Like the cLMA it consists of an airway tube with a silicone mask at the end, designed to sit over and seal the larynx. There are many differences from the cLMA. The airway tube is rigid, shorter and wider than the cLMA (allowing passage of an 8.0 mm tracheal tube). At the proximal end of the airway tube is a metal handle, which allows insertion, and manipulation, of the device without placing fingers in the patient's mouth. Within the airway tube, close to the distal end is a v-shaped groove that centralizes the tracheal tube as it exits the airway. At the distal end of the airway tube in place of the bars of the cLMA is an 'epiglottic elevator' (Figure 6.3). This is a firm silicone bar attached only at its superior end, which is elevated by the tracheal tube as it exits the airway. The ILMA needs a minimum of 2.0 cm mouth opening to allow insertion. Sizes 3–5 are available.

The ILMA is provided with a reusable tracheal tube and a silicone tube stabilizer. The tracheal tubes (size 7.0, 7.5 or 8.0 mm) are wire-reinforced and have a bullet nosed, soft silicone tip. The 15 mm connector is removable. The tube has markings to indicate correct orientation of the tip and the point at which the tube tip exits the ILMA during insertion. The tubes are designed to reduce laryngeal trauma during blind placement and have been shown to perform better than conventional tubes.

There are three stages to tracheal intubation with the ILMA:

1 *ILMA placement*: With the head and neck in the neutral position, the ILMA is inserted with the

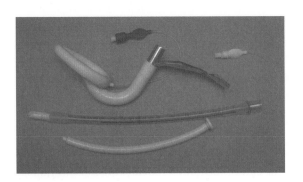

Figure 6.2 The ILMA kit.

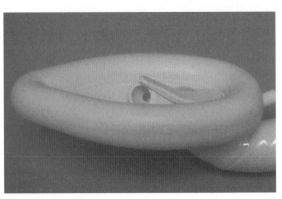

Figure 6.3 Epiglottic elevator.

handle parallel to the chest. It is then advanced along the hard palate while rotating in the arc of the airway. The ILMA is inserted until the device tip reaches the cricopharyngeus muscle and resistance is felt. The cuff is inflated and the anaesthetic circuit attached. The handle is used to optimize the position of the ILMA. The aim being to find the position in which ventilation is easiest with lowest resistance, correlating with optimum positioning of the ILMA over the laryngeal inlet.

2 *Tracheal tube placement*: The anaesthetic circuit is detached while maintaining ILMA position. The well-lubricated tracheal tube is then inserted, with the black line of the tube lying posteriorly, to correctly orientate the tube bevel. After passing beyond the distal end the tracheal tube may need rotating to enter the trachea (resistance to insertion indicates a need for repositioning). The anaesthetic circuit is attached, the tracheal tube cuff inflated and correct placement of the tracheal tube confirmed with auscultation and capnography.

3 *Removal of the ILMA*: The tracheal tube connector is removed, the ILMA cuff deflated and the ILMA withdrawn. The tracheal tube is maintained in place by placing an obturator into the ILMA, which allows stabilization of tracheal tube position while removing the ILMA. The tracheal tube connector is once again attached and tube position reconfirmed. As this technique is a form of 'blind tracheal intubation' (the larynx is not seen during intubation) it is important to confirm tube position and exclude endobronchial intubation.

The main criticism of this method of intubation is that it is 'blind'. Techniques using the fibrescope are increasingly popular. A 'tube first' or 'scope first' technique may be used. Using the tube first approach the tracheal tube is advanced until the epiglottic elevator is lifted out of the way, before passing a fibrescope to guide the tube into the larynx. In the scope first technique the fibrescope (inside the tracheal tube) is advanced into the larynx with the tracheal tube held more proximally, before railroading over the fibrescope. The ILMA may also be used with a lighted stylet such as the trachlight to guide intubation.

The ILMA may be used for elective or emergency intubation. The blind technique should not be used in patients with pharyngeal or oesophageal pathology. The blind technique requires manual ventilation via the ILMA and it should be remembered that the ILMA, like the cLMA, does not protect against aspiration, so the technique should be avoided where there is increased risk of regurgitation. When necessary the ILMA may be placed in awake patients after the application of topical anaesthesia.

Comparisons with the cLMA have shown that the airway seal achieved with the ILMA is higher than with the cLMA. The view of the larynx is poorer with the ILMA than the cLMA, with the larynx visible in some 10–15% fewer cases. The mucosal pressure exerted by the ILMA is greater and minor pharyngolaryngeal morbidity greater than with the cLMA. It is recommended that the ILMA is removed after intubation unless there is a specific indication to leave it in place. Intubation with the ILMA causes the same haemodynamic responses as conventional tracheal intubation.

Early evaluation in patients with normal airways showed successful intubation in 149 of 150 patients including 13 with known difficulty. Fewer manoeuvres were needed in those with predicted or known difficult airways. Further evaluations have shown intubation success of 93–100% within three attempts. First time success with a blind technique is between 72% and 80%. In a series of 254 cases with known difficulties with intubation, tracheal intubation was achieved in 76% on the first attempt and in 97% after up to five attempts. Overall success was 96% using a blind technique and 100% using a fibrescope-guided technique.

There is controversy over the use of the ILMA in routine anaesthesia. While some would consider use of the ILMA is an acceptable routine method for tracheal intubation, others cite the increase in minor complications, in particular sore throat and hoarseness as reasons to avoid its use. As the ILMA has a learning curve, of approximately 20 cases, this makes training potentially problematic. Controversy was increased by the report of a death due to oesophageal perforation after elective use of the ILMA. A blind technique was used and the patient had an oesophageal pouch. For training purposes patient consent is necessary, where the technique is not a routine part of the anaesthetist's practice, a fibrescope-guided technique is advisable and pharyngeal or oesophageal pathology are contra-indications to ILMA use.

The ILMA has a role in tracheal intubation in the trauma patient both in and out of hospital. It is designed to be inserted with the head and neck in the neutral position and upper cervical movement during its use with in line stabilization is minimal. Use of a fibrescope-guided technique increases success during in line stabilization. A hard collar and application of cricoid pressure both prevent correct placement of the ILMA.

The ILMA (with tracheal tube and stabilizer) costs approximately £300 and is reusable 40 times. A single use version is due to be available in 2004.

ProSeal LMA

The (PLMA™) was introduced in the UK in January 2001 (Figure 6.4). It is designed by Dr Archie Brain, is based on the cLMA and is designed to improve performance and safety during controlled ventilation. Modifications include a softer, larger bowl, a posterior extension of the cuff, a drainage tube running parallel to the airway tube and an integral bite block. When correctly placed, the PLMA lies with the drain tube in continuity with the oesophagus and the airway tube in continuity with the trachea. This allows functional separation of the alimentary and respiratory tracts. The drain tube vents gas leaking from the mask into the oesophagus and prevents gastric distension, allows passage of an orogastric tube (OGT) and vents regurgitated stomach contents. The changes in the shape of the PLMA bowl improve the seal with the larynx. The drain tube allows early diagnosis or misplacement of the PLMA, which is not always possible with the cLMA.

Sizes 3–5 are available and sizes 1.5–2.5 will soon be available. Sizes below 3 do not have the posterior extension of the cuff. Size selection is as for other LMA devices. The PLMA is supplied with a cuff-deflator, which is recommended to aid complete deflation of the device and flattening of the tip, before insertion. Complete deflation lessens deflection of the epiglottis or entry of the tip into the glottis.

A greater depth of anaesthesia is required for insertion of the PLMA than the cLMA. The PLMA may be inserted with or without the supplied introducer (Figure 6.5). Without the introducer the technique is the same to that for the cLMA and with the introducer is as for the ILMA. There is no convincing evidence that one method is preferable to the other. Particular care must be taken when removing the

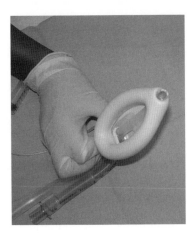

Figure 6.4 Proseal.

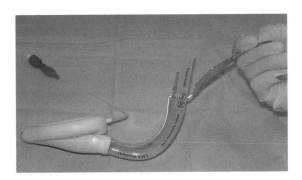

Figure 6.5 Proseal with introducer.

introducer to avoid dental damage. After insertion the cuff is inflated and the manufacturers recommend inflation to an intracuff pressure of 60 cmH$_2$O. An OGT can be passed through the drain tube when indicated. This should be well lubricated and not refrigerated. If there is difficulty with insertion the PLMA may be placed by railroading the drain tube over a gum elastic bougie intentionally placed in the oesophagus.

An important feature of the PLMA is that the drain tube allows early diagnosis of misplacement of the device. This in turn allows early correction of position and optimal function. It is unclear whether the PLMA is prone to misplacement more commonly than the cLMA, but diagnosis is easier. If the PLMA is placed too proximally ventilated air is vented via the drain tube. If the tip is placed in the glottis, venting of gas occurs similarly but airway obstruction may also occur. If the PLMA tip folds over during insertion the functionality of the drain tube is lost. This misplacement is readily diagnosed by inability to pass an OGT to the tip of the PLMA. Gel or soap placed over the proximal drain tube orifice may assist in diagnosing these misplacements and confirming correct function.

Successful insertion and ventilation rates of above 95% can be achieved. First time insertion rates are somewhat lower and time taken for insertion longer than for the cLMA although the relevant studies may be biased by researchers previous experience with the cLMA.

Airway seal pressure with the PLMA is approximately 30 cmH$_2$O (cLMA 20 cmH$_2$O) and exceeds 40 cmH$_2$O in about 20% of cases. Results are similar whether the PLMA is used in paralysed or non-paralysed patients. The improved seal allows successful ventilation in cases where this would not be achieved with the cLMA.

The PLMA improves the success of controlled ventilation compared to the cLMA. Design and performance features of the PLMA make it likely that its use reduces the likelihood of gastric inflation and protects from aspiration if regurgitation

occurs. There is robust experimental and clinical evidence to support this belief, but it is unproven and probably unprovable.

OGT passage is successful in >90% of cases at the first attempt. Ease of passage of an OGT correlates with fibreoptic position of the PLMA over the larynx. Where there is doubt over correct positioning of the PLMA an OGT should be passed and if this fails the PLMA should be resited.

Extended uses of the PLMA include the use for laparoscopic surgery, selected open abdominal surgery, in the obese, those with minor gastro-oesophageal reflux, as an adjunct for difficult intubation and as a rescue device after failed intubation. Areas of interest outside the operating theatre include use in intensive care unit (ICU) and during resuscitation. Most of these areas have not been adequately explored yet.

The PLMA may used 40 times.

Cost is £100, which includes introducer tool and deflator device.

Combitube

The combitube was developed in Austria by Dr Frass in the 1980s. It resembles the oesophageal obturator airway with dual lumens. It consists of a double lumen tube with dual cuffs and depth of insertion markings to aid positioning. There are two sizes (37F and 41F) for small and larger adults. The combitube is not recommended for patients of <4 foot height.

The distal portion of the tube resembles a cuffed tracheal tube. This lumen of the combitube can be inserted into the trachea and is then indeed used as a tracheal tube with the breathing circuit attached to the 'tracheo-esophageal tube'. When the distal tube is inserted into the oesophagus the distal cuff is inflated to occlude the oesophagus. A larger proximal cuff lies at the level of the base of the tongue. This high volume cuff is inflated to stabilize the tube position and occlude the oropharynx. Ventilation is then achieved through the 'pharyngeal tube' via ventilation holes sited between the two cuffs. In this position, delayed expiration through the ventilation holes may lead to development of positive end expiratory presssure (PEEP) and may improve oxygenation.

There are two distinct insertion techniques. During elective use the device should be used with a laryngoscope and placed under direct vision (the site the distal tube is placed may depend on training needs). In the emergency situation the combitube is placed blindly. The head and neck may be in the neutral or flexed position but the sniffing position is actively avoided. The anterior mandible and tongue are lifted anteriorly by gripping these between the operator's fingers, while the combitube is advanced. In contrast to cLMA insertion the combitube is advanced along the tongue (not the hard palate). The volumes of air inserted into the cuffs are: distal 5–15 ml and proximal 85–150 ml (reduced initially to 40 ml in elective cases).

The attraction of the design is that whether the distal tube is placed in the trachea or the oesophagus, ventilation is possible. When placed in the oesophagus the distal tube may offer protection from aspiration of regurgitant matter. A criticism of the design is potential complexity and confusion in its use. The use of capnography will reduce potentially fatal misdiagnosis.

Clinical reports show the combitube can be very successful when used as a rescue device after failed tracheal intubation. During blind placement, the distal tube is placed in the oesophagus in approximately 98% of cases. The use of the combitube during routine anaesthesia is highly controversial. There is no strong argument for its use over other available SADs. The combitube is a single-use device and some three times more expensive than equivalent devices. There have been reports of high incidences of mucosal trauma with routine use. On balance the combitube cannot be recommended for use for airway management during routine anaesthesia.

Traditionally there have been two sizes (41F and 37F). The 37F size is most appropriate for the majority of patients. More recently the combitube has been modified, including a reduction in size, in an attempt to reduce the trauma associated with

its use. The pharyngeal ventilation holes have been enlarged to assist access to the trachea when the combitube is placed in the oesophagus, thus allowing tracheal suction or exchange to a more definitive airway. A paediatric version (26F) has been reported in abstracts for use in children between the heights of 3 and 4 feet.

The combitube remains significantly less popular in the UK than in North America. It is part of the American, Canadian and UK difficult airway management algorithms and International Liaison Committee on Resuscitation (ILCOR) recommendations for airway control during cardiopulmonary resuscitation.

The combitube is for single use only and costs approximately £30.

Other devices

Laryngeal tube
The Laryngeal Tube (LT®) is designed for use during spontaneous or controlled ventilation. It consists of a slim airway tube with a small balloon cuff attached at the tip and a larger asymmetric balloon cuff at the middle part of the tube both of which are inflated by a single pilot tube. Markings assist correct depth of insertion. Cuff inflation creates a seal and ventilation occurs through orifices between the cuffs. The cuffs are inflated to a pressure of 60–70 cmH$_2$O. Five sizes are available intended for all patient ages and the LT is designed to be reused up to 50 times.

The LT was modified twice between 2001 and 2003. Most available trials have used earlier versions of the LT rather than the currently available device. Initial evaluations with the original device reported very low success rates during spontaneous ventilation. More recent studies suggest high success rates for insertion (>95%) and good airway seal pressure (approximately 28 cmH$_2$O). The slim profile of the LT allows easy insertion with little mouth opening and the device causes minimal airway trauma. There is no published work studying whether the lower cuff protects against aspiration of regurgitated stomach contents. Trials with the current LT have shown similar performance to the cLMA during controlled ventilation, but requiring more manipulations and poorer performance than the PLMA.

LT Sonda

The *LT Sonda* (LTS®) is a modification of the LT, which differs in having a drain tube (which runs posterior to the airway tube), to allow gastric tube placement and prevent gastric inflation during ventilation.

Airway management device

The *Airway Management Device* (AMD™) superficially resembles the LT with a distal and superficial cuff designed to straddle and isolate the larynx. The cuffs are inflated by separate pilot balloons. The distal balloon has a conduit designed to allow oesophageal suction. There are three (adult) sizes. The AMD was modified in 2001 and is designed to be reused up to 40 times. Two studies, performed with the currently available device, show a failure rate of the device of 15–20%. Despite relatively few cases of AMD use reported in the literature (<300) two cases of regurgitation and one of aspiration are cause for concern. On the basis of the available evidence the AMD appears to have little role in routine anaesthesia.

Pharyngeal Airway xpress

The *Pharyngeal Airway xpress* (PAx™) is a single use device consisting of a wide bore semi-rigid airway tube attached to a large 'head' of silicone gills, distal to a ventilation orifice and a proximal cuff. The gills deform during insertion and are designed to stabilize position. Only one size is available and it is suitable for patients weighing >45 kg. It was modified twice in 2001–2002 and again in 2003. Two studies of early versions of the PAx report high incidences of trauma and sore throat after its use. More recent small studies are more encouraging but there is inadequate information published on the current version of the device.

Cobra Perilaryngeal airway

The *Cobra Perilaryngeal airway* (CobraPLA™) is a new single use wide bore airway with distal obturator and proximal cuff. The distal end (somewhat resembling a cobra head, so lending the name to the device) consists of a firm scalloped plastic head designed to sit in and seal the hypopharynx, with the anterior surface abutting the larynx. In this respect it differs from most other 'obturator/ cuff devices', as the distal tip lies proximal to the oesophageal inlet. The anterior surface consists of a grille of soft bars, soft enough to allow instrumentation of the larynx, through which gas exchange takes place. A proximal balloon elevates the tongue base and seals the oropharynx. Multiple sizes for infant to large adult are available. The CobraPLA is designed for spontaneous and controlled ventilation. There is little published experience with the CobraPLA and in particular its safety with regard to aspiration. What evidence there is suggests insertion is successful in 80% on the first attempt, airway seal is approximately 25 cmH$_2$O and minor morbidity is of similar order to that for the cLMA.

Streamlined Liner of the Pharynx Airway

The *Streamlined Liner of the Pharynx Airway* (SLIPA) is a single use device likely to be launched in 2004. It is of novel design: a soft plastic blow-moulded airway with the shape mimicking a 'pressurized pharynx'. In appearance the SLIPA slightly resembles a boot. It has no cuff and at least six sizes are likely. The hollow device has the capacity to accommodate 30–70 ml of fluid and the manufacturers suggest that this may offer protection against aspiration, should regurgitation occur. There is currently no clinical data to confirm this. Early cohort and comparative trials by the inventor have shown satisfactory insertion rates and performance. Larger independent trials are needed.

Key points

- Airway obstruction is likely to occur at induction of anaesthesia and will lead to hypoxia if not recognized and reversed.
- Airway obstruction is caused by posterior movement of the soft palate, tongue and glottic opening. Manoeuvres that counteract obstruction

include positioning in the sniffing position, chin lift and jaw thrust.

- Airway adjuncts (Guedel and nasal airways) clear the airway of soft tissue obstruction and improve the efficiency of bag and face mask ventilation.
- Supra-glottic airways are frequently used for elective surgery and aim to provide a clear, safe airway requiring minimal manipulation.
- The LMA is the gold standard at present.
- Many available supra-glottic airways have limited evaluation before being introduced to the market.
- All supra-glottic airways may lead to downfolding of the epiglottis and laryngeal obstruction. Different airways seek different solutions to this problem.
- No supra-glottic airway is proven to protect against pulmonary aspiration of regurgitated stomach contents.
- The performance of different supra-glottic airways during controlled vs. spontaneous ventilation, and with regard to positioning over the larynx, airway seal and minor airway trauma differs considerably.
- A major benefit of single use devices over reusable devices is yet to be demonstrated.

Further reading

Boidin MP. Airway patency in the unconscious patient. *Br J Anaesth* 1985; **57**: 306–308.

Calder I, Picard J, Chapman M, O'Sullevan C, Crockard HA. Mouth opening – a new angle. *Anesthesiology* 2003; **99**: 799–801.

Cook TM. Spoilt for choice? New supraglottic airways. *Anaesthesia* 2003; **58**: 107–110.

Defalque RJ, Weight AJ. Who invented the jaw thrust? *Anesthesiology* 2003; **99**: 1463–1464.

Grady DM, McHardy F, Wong J *et al.* Pharyngolaryngeal morbidity with the laryngeal mask airway in spontaneously breathing patients: does size matter? *Anesthesiology* 2001; **94**: 760–766.

Nandi PR, Charlesworth CH, Taylor SJ, Nunn JF, Doré CJ. Effect of general anaesthesia on the pharynx. *Br J Anaesth* 1991; **66**:157–162.

Yarrow S, Hare J, Robinson KN. Recent trends in tracheal intubation: a retrospective analysis. *Anaesthesia* 2003; **58**: 1019–1022.

V. Mitchell & A. Patel

The placement of a cuffed tube in the trachea offers the highest level of airway maintenance and protection, and is often the most appropriate route for provision of mechanical ventilation. This chapter concentrates on characteristics of the tube rather than the means of inserting it into the trachea.

History

Intubation of the trachea via the larynx was first described by Macewen of Glasgow in 1878 but only began to gain popularity in the 1920s with the description of blind nasal intubation by Rowbotham and Magill. This technique was quick, accurate and gained early control of the airway. Magill made his own tubes, which he cut from lengths of rubber tubing, bevelling the ends and smoothing the tips with sandpaper before storing them in a biscuit tin to attain the desired curve.

Various materials are used in the construction of tracheal tubes and each has its own properties (Table 7.1). Traditional mineralized red rubber tubes are still in use but began to be replaced with plastic tubes from the 1950s. Plastic tubes are made of polyvinyl chloride or polyurethane, offer a number of advantages and are widely used. Silicone tubes are available but less widely used as they are more expensive to manufacture. Polyvinyl chloride and polyurethane tubes may be siliconized as part of the manufacturing process. In the past, some materials used in the manufacture of tracheal tubes have shown evidence of tissue toxicity. Implant testing (IT) or cell culture are mandatory to exclude toxicity when a new material is used, without it the device cannot be marketed.

Table 7.1 Characteristics of materials from which tubes are manufactured

Material	Characteristics
Mineralized rubber	Soft and springy
	Can be sterilized and reused
	May become blocked with inspissated secretions
	Opaque
	Rubber fatigues over time and may kink
	Cuff characteristics: high pressure, low volume
	Cuffs tend to inflate irregularly and may herniate
	Cannot be used in patients with latex allergy
Plastic (PVC or polyurethane)	Non-irritant
	Single use only
	Inexpensive to manufacture to a high standard
	Easy to sterilize during manufacture
	Thermoplastic – softens when warmed
	Can be transparent, opaque or siliconized
	Less tendency to kink than rubber
	Stiffer than rubber or silicone
	Less elasticity than rubber
Silicone	Soft
	Floppy
	Can be autoclaved
	Expensive to manufacture

Design

Standard tubes have a preformed curve that approximately conforms to the anatomy of the pharynx and which aids insertion and resists kinking of the tube *in situ*. The cross section is round as both oval and ellipses are more prone to kinking. The distal tip is cut at an oblique angle (bevelled) so that the aperture opens to the left if the tube is held in the right hand. The angle of the bevel is $38° ± 10°$. The left-facing bevel allows visualization of the tip of the tube as it passes through the cords when introduced with the right hand. The shape of the distal portion of the tube may vary (Figure 7.1).

Some tubes have a window or Murphy Eye cut into the wall opposite the bevel. This provides an alternative route for gas flow should the bevel become obstructed by impaction against the tracheal wall. It also provides an inadvertent and unwelcome route for fibrescopes, tube exchangers and percutaneous tracheostomies, and means that the cuff cannot be as close to the tip of the tube. The nomenclature is confusing since some authors refer to tubes with a Murphy eye as Murphy tubes and those without as Magill tubes and others refer to all standard curved tubes as Magill tubes whether or not they have a Murphy eye. The tube may also have an inflatable cuff which, when inflated, seals the space between the tube and the tracheal wall.

Markings

Various markings are seen on the tracheal tube or packaging (Table 7.2). Reference lines, rings or coloured areas are sometimes used to help position the tube with respect to the vocal cords. Materials from which tracheal tubes are manufactured must be tested for biological safety. This is generally established with IT in rabbit paravertebral muscle.

Until 1996 tubes were marked with a test number, F-29 or IT on a tube denoting that the material from which it was made had been tested and shown no evidence of toxicity. Currently, any product which is marketed in the European Union (EU) must meet the requirement of all relevant EU Directives including biological safety in order to carry the Confirmite Europeene (CE) mark, and in the US the Food and Drug Administration (FDA) does not allow products to be sold unless biological safety has been established. The CE mark is carried on the tube packaging.

Sizing

Tubes are sized by the internal diameter in millimetres. Due to variations in wall thickness there are significant differences between the external diameters of tubes of the same size (Figure 7.2). Conventional wisdom suggests the use of the widest diameter tube

---

Table 7.2 Markings on tracheal tubes

- Tube size in internal diameter in millimetres
- The outside diameter for size 6 and smaller
- The words oral or nasal or oral/nasal
- Name or trademark of the supplier
- Radio-opaque longitudinal line (may be of barium sulphate which increases risk of laser fire by reducing temperature at which ignition of the tube occurs)
- Distance from tip in centimetres marked on the wall
- Do not reuse or single use only if disposable

Additional markings may be added. Reference lines, rings or coloured areas are sometimes used to help position the tube with respect to the vocal cords.
Compliance with CE or International Organization for Standardization (ISO) regulations is marked on the packaging.

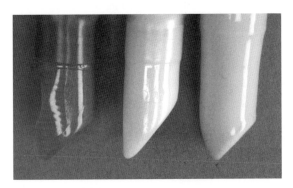

Figure 7.1 Distal tips of various tubes: from left Sheridan reinforced, Portex nasal, ILMA tube.

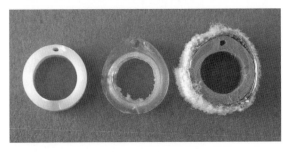

Figure 7.2 All tubes have the same internal diameter: from left microlaryngeal, reinforced, Sheridan laser.

that will pass easily through the cords (or the cricoid ring in a child). Both large and small tubes have a number of advantages and disadvantages (Table 7.3). A large tube reduces resistance to gas flow and work of breathing. In conditions of laminar flow, resistance is inversely proportional to the fourth power of the radius according to the Hagen–Poiseuille equation. Even though flow is often turbulent *in vivo*, each millimetre decrease in tube diameter increases tube resistance by between 25% and 100%. An increase in the work of breathing parallels the increase in resistance as tube size is reduced, a 1 mm decrease in tube diameter increases the work of breathing by up to 150% depending on the minute volume.

Traditionally, in British anaesthesia, an 8.0 mm tube was placed in adult female patients and a 9.0 mm tube in males. However, the necessity for these large sizes has been challenged. Smaller tubes are easier to insert because the view of the laryngeal inlet is less likely to be obscured during passage of the tube through the cords at direct laryngoscopy. There is less laryngeal trauma on insertion and for the duration of intubation and there is a lower incidence of sore throat. For provision of anaesthesia, physiologically normal adult patients can be managed perfectly well with size 6.0 and 7.0 mm tubes for both spontaneous respiration and mechanical ventilation. In paediatric practice it is usual to place the largest uncuffed tube which will permit a small leak and various formulae exist to indicate the likely size for a particular paediatric patient (Table 7.4).

Length

The tube length from the tip is shown on the outside in centimetres. The correct insertion depth is important to avoid the morbidity of endobronchial

Table 7.3 Comparison of small and large tracheal tubes

	Small tubes	Large tubes
Advantages	Easier to insert Less laryngeal trauma Lower incidence of sore throat	Lower work of breathing in spontaneously breathing patients Tracheal suctioning is easier
Disadvantages	Increased airway resistance Excessive cuff volumes Auto-PEEP Difficult to suction Difficult fibreoptic endoscopy	Harder to insert More laryngeal trauma Infolding of cuff may allow tracheal soiling

Table 7.4 Recommended tube sizes in children

Age	Weight (kg)	Size (id)	Length (cm) Oral	Nasal
Neonate	2–4	2.5–3.5	10–12	15
1–6 months	4–6	3.5–4	12–14	15
6–12 months	6–10	3.5–4.0	14–16	15
1–3 years	10–15	4.0–4.5	16–18	16
4–6 years	15–20	4.5–5.5	18–20	17
7–10 years	25–35	5.5–6.0	20–22	18–20

Below 8–10 years uncuffed tubes should be used.

Tube size (internal diameter (id)) in children $= \dfrac{\text{Age in years}}{2} + 2\frac{1}{2}$ or $\dfrac{\text{age in years}}{4} + 4$

Oral tube length (cm) $= 12 + \dfrac{\text{Age in years}}{2}$

Nasal tube length (cm) $= 15 + \dfrac{\text{Age in years}}{2}$

placement, inflation of the cuff within the larynx or accidental extubation during the procedure. The position of the tube tip in relation to the carina will be altered by gross movements of the head with head/neck extension causing withdrawal of the tube. Ideally, the tip of an uncuffed tube should be in the mid-trachea so that inadvertent extubation or endobronchial migration are minimized. For a neonate with trachea length 4 cm, the tip should be 2 cm below the vocal cords. With a cuffed tube, it is important that the insertion depth is sufficient to avoid inflating the cuff within the larynx itself. Many tubes carry depth markers (usually one or two solid black lines) which indicate the correct depth when the markers are placed at the level of the glottis. Depth of insertion is generally referred to by the centimetre marking at the teeth or corner of the mouth.

Cuffs

The cuff and inflation system consists of an inflation lumen in the wall of the tube, an external inflation tube, a pilot balloon and a self-sealing inflation valve. Cuffed tubes are generally used in adult practice to seal the airway to protect it from soiling from above and to prevent gas leaks. Cuff pressure is transmitted to the tracheal wall at the points of contact and this is termed the lateral wall pressure. To prevent aspiration, lateral wall pressure should exceed the maximum hydrostatic pressure that can be generated by a column of liquid (saliva, vomitus or blood) above the cuff. This hydrostatic pressure depends on the vertical distance from the upper part of the mouth and changes with the position of the patient. This distance is approximately 10–15 cm in the supine patient and 15–20 cm in the erect, necessitating pressures of 20 cmH$_2$O in the supine position and 25 cmH$_2$O in the erect position. The lateral wall pressure cannot be measured directly and is not necessarily predictable from the intracuff pressure. Obstruction to tracheal mucosal blood flow occurs at a lateral wall pressure above 30 cmH$_2$O and total occlusion occurs at 50 cmH$_2$O.

A high cuff pressure reduces the risk of aspiration but at the expense of high lateral wall pressures causing sore throat, mucosal inflammation progressing

to ulceration, cartilaginous destruction and tracheal stenosis. Three factors contribute to the extent of cuff-induced tracheal damage:

- cuff characteristics
- pressure regulation
- inflation technique and medium.

Cuff characteristics

Cuffs may be categorized by their volume and pressure characteristics into two broad groups (Figure 7.3) with their own characteristics (Table 7.5).

Low volume, high pressure

Early red rubber tubes had a small resting diameter, a low residual volume and low compliance. A high intracuff pressure is required to achieve a seal within the trachea. There is a small area of contact within the trachea and the cuff distends and deforms the trachea to a circular shape. In this sort

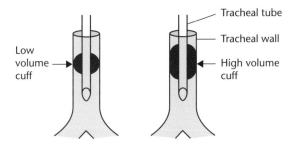

Figure 7.3 The two types of cuff. Difference in seal area with high volume low pressure and low volume high pressure cuffs.

Table 7.5 Advantages of high volume, low pressure tubes

- Low tracheal wall pressure at occluding pressure spares mucosal perfusion
- Cuff inflates evenly on all sides giving a large area of seal
- Tube stabilized in the centre of the trachea and tip is not pushed against tracheal wall
- Wide margin of error in selecting tube size allowing smaller tube and reducing laryngeal damage
- Redundancy of the cuff permits small up and down movements of the tube without tube displacement so abrasive movement of the cuff against the trachea is reduced

of cuff most of the pressure is needed to overcome cuff wall compliance (i.e. to stretch the cuff), so the pressure exerted against the tracheal wall is lower than intracuff pressure but the relationship between the two is non-linear. The use of a tube diameter close to that of the trachea permits low volume inflation and relative tracheal mucosal protection but increases the potential for laryngeal damage because the diameter of the tube is greater and trauma to laryngeal structures during insertion or friction injury to cords while the tube is in place is more likely. Recognition of the deleterious effects of early cuffs led to the development of high volume, low pressure cuffs in the 1970s.

High volume, low pressure cuffs

Modern tracheal tube cuffs have a large resting volume and diameter and a thin compliant wall which allows a seal to be achieved without stretching the cuff wall. When inflated, the thin, floppy cuff adapts itself to the tracheal contour. In this type of tube, cuff size is important. Intracuff pressure reflects lateral wall pressure unless the resting cuff circumference is less than tracheal circumference, in which case it will be stretched beyond its residual volume at seal point and will behave like a high pressure cuff.

The optimal cuff is therefore, sufficiently large to effect a seal before being inflated to its residual volume.

Despite these apparent advantages, there is little evidence of benefit in clinical anaesthesia when high volume cuffs are compared to their low volume, high pressure predecessors. This may be due to the fact that although the pressure on the tracheal mucosa may be lower with high volume cuffs, the area of contact is greater. The large, floppy cuff may also obscure the view at direct laryngoscopy increasing the likelihood of trauma on insertion, and once residual volume is exceeded, a 2–3 ml inflation increment is sufficient to cause an exponential rise in cuff pressure resulting in unsafe lateral wall pressures.

Pressure regulating cuffs

Several cuff systems designed to minimize intra-cuff pressure changes are commercially available

(Figures 7.4–7.6) but none has demonstrated significant clinical benefit. The Brandt™ cuff system pilot balloon allows re-diffusion of nitrous oxide so that a low pressure seal is maintained. The Lanz™

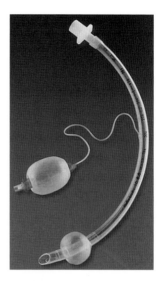

Figure 7.4 Brandt tube.

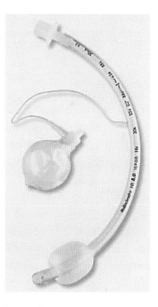

Figure 7.5 Lanz tube.

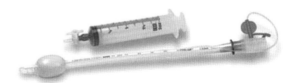

Figure 7.6 Fome-cuff.

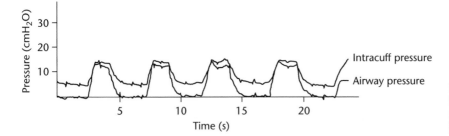

Figure 7.7 Linkage of intracuff with airway pressure (intermittent positive pressure ventilation).

cuff system consists of a compliant pilot balloon inside a transparent sheath with a pressure regulating valve between them and provides a constant cuff pressure below 3.4 kPa. The valve allows rapid gas flow from the balloon to the cuff but only slow flow from the cuff to the balloon. This prevents leakage of gas when airway pressure rises rapidly in inspiration but prevents cuff pressure rising during nitrous oxide anaesthesia.

The Smith Portex soft seal cuff claims to be less permeable to nitrous oxide limiting the intraoperative rise in cuff pressure and the Smith Portex Fome-Cuf™ tube features a polyurethane foam filled cuff which exerts a table lateral wall pressure which is independent of inflation medium and temperature.

Pressure regulation

Measurements of cuff pressure are complicated by the fact that the intracuff pressure may not represent the lateral wall pressure especially in a low volume, high pressure tube where much of the intracuff pressure is needed to overcome the compliance of the cuff. Despite this, the measurement of cuff pressure is clinically useful in avoiding excessive mucosal pressure since cuff pressure *always* exceeds lateral wall pressure. In addition, cuff pressure varies with the respiratory cycle (Figure 7.7). In the spontaneously breathing patient airway pressure and cuff pressure are negative during inspiration. During controlled ventilation, positive pressure is applied to the distal portion of the cuff during inspiration and the air in the cuff is compressed until intracuff pressure equals airway pressure. Several methods have been used for continuous or intermittent measurement of cuff pressure, the most useful being a commercially available cuff pressure monitor (Figure 7.8).

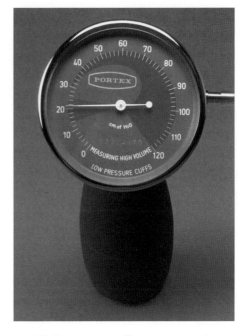

Figure 7.8 Portex intracuff pressure monitor: green segment indicates desirable range.

Table 7.6 Cuff pressures using seal technique for inflation with different inflation media

Cuff pressure to seal (mmHg)	Air	Saline	O_2/N_2O 'GasMix'
Mean	35.3	22.5	27
Range	9–119	8–41	2–53
SD	31.61	11.27	20.7

Inflation technique and medium

When cuff inflation is carried out using the leak technique, the cuff pressure obtained varies widely (Table 7.6). If inflation is carried out with air, cuff pressure will increase significantly during nitrous

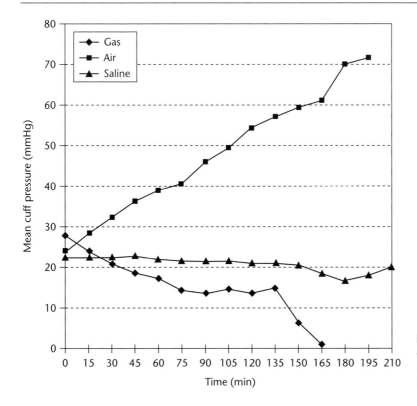

Figure 7.9 Changes in tracheal cuff pressure during anaesthesia with N_2O with either air, saline or O_2/N_2O mix in cuff.

oxide anaesthesia as nitrous oxide diffuses into the cuff along a concentration gradient (Figure 7.9). The diffusion of oxygen into the cuff and expansion of air as it warms to body temperature may also contribute to a pressure increase.

Saline provides stable cuff pressures but is more difficult to use than air. Saline is more viscous than air or gas and the cuff must be inflated more slowly than usual to allow time for equilibration of pressure throughout the system. The elasticity of the cuff tends to force saline back into the pilot balloon when filling pressure is discontinued, resulting in a drop in intracuff pressure if the process is completed too quickly. Saline is not suitable for reusable tube cuffs as they will explode when autoclaved.

If a mixture of inspired gases containing nitrous oxide is used to inflate the cuff, deflation of the cuff may occur. The pressure inside the cuff is above atmospheric pressure and the intracuff partial pressure of nitrous oxide is greater than that of the inspired gas. Nitrous oxide diffuses out of the cuff along a pressure gradient and the cuff may deflate.

Connectors

Tracheal tubes are attached to the breathing system via tapered male to female 15 mm ISO connectors. The male connector fits the tube via a tapered cone whose diameter is slightly larger than the tube ensuring a secure connection. The tube adaptor (catheter mount) or breathing circuit house the female part of the system with an internal diameter of 15 mm and an outer diameter of 22 mm. An 8.5 mm diameter connector is available for paediatric tubes. Non-ISO connectors such as metal Magill or flexibend connectors are now rarely used.

Special tubes

Polar

Commonly known as RAE tubes (after the designers Ring-Adair-Elwyn, Salt Lake City), polar tubes are preformed so that their ISO connector is distant from the mouth or the nose (Figure 7.10). A bulky angled connector and catheter mount are avoided and the tube can be fixed securely in place with strapping on the chin or forehead with little or no risk of kinking or dislodgement. Both oral and nasal tubes are available in either north- or south-facing pattern with the 'facing' indicating that the tube is preformed to be directed cephalad (north) or caudad (south). North-facing polar nasal tubes (Figure 7.11) are particularly useful in head and neck surgery where access to the oral cavity is required. The main disadvantages are with the fixed length of the intraoral or intranasal section and difficulty with suctioning through a long, tightly curved tube. They can be converted to conventional tubes by cutting the tube at its bend and reinserting the ISO connector.

Armoured or reinforced

Standard tubes kink when twisted or compressed. The walls of armoured tubes contain a spiral of

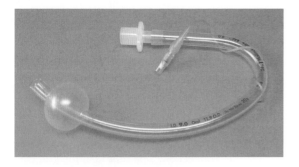

Figure 7.10 South-facing oral RAE tube.

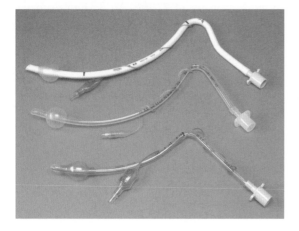

Figure 7.11 Nasal, north-facing polar tubes.

metal wire or nylon (Figure 7.12) to prevent kinking or occlusion of the tube when the head or neck are moved. The reinforcement allows the tube to be made of a more elastic material which makes it less traumatic but more difficult to insert as it tends to be floppy with no preformed shape. It is preferable to have the reinforcement welded to the ISO connector to avoid the vulnerable junction of tube and connector, which is liable to kink. The reinforced tubes supplied for use with the intubating laryngeal mask airway (ILMA) are the exception to this rule as the connector must be removed during the passage of the tube through the ILMA.

The external diameter of armoured tubes is greater than ordinary tubes of the same size due to their thicker walls and the tubes are designed for oral or nasal intubation so they are relatively long and inadvertent endobronchial intubation may occur if insufficient attention is paid to positioning. There are circumferential markers to indicate the correct position for the vocal cords. Armoured tubes cannot be cut and must be fixed in place with adhesive tapes. There are two hazards particular to the use of an armoured tube for oral intubation. As there is no preformed curve there is more potential for longitudinal movement of the tube and complete occlusion may occur if the patient bites on the tube as the reinforcing wire can be permanently deformed. If an armoured tube has been used for an oral intubation it is usual to insert a Guedel airway adjacent to the tube to avoid this complication and to stabilize it.

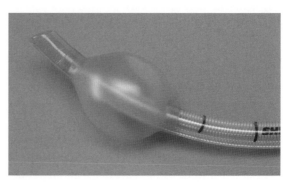

Figure 7.12 Armoured tube: note wire spiral in wall and insertion depth markings.

Laser tubes

Standard and microlaryngoscopy tubes are unsuitable for laser airway procedures due to the high energies contained within the laser beam. Three components (Figure 7.13) are required simultaneously

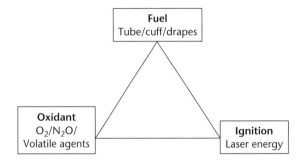

Figure 7.13 Laser fire triangle. All three components of the triangle must be present for an airway fire to occur. If one component is removed (e.g. no plastic tube or fuel source) the situation is safe. If all three components are present to some extent during laser surgery, it is essential to minimize oxidant source by using the lowest FiO_2 to maintain SpO_2 using air as the diluent.

for a laser-induced fire, and a plastic or red rubber tube provides the fuel element. When combined with high concentrations of oxygen, the tube will quickly incinerate within the airway causing fatal damage. Laser tubes have laser resistant properties (so that the laser energy coming into contact with the fuel source is much reduced) but the tubes may ignite with sustained laser energy strikes of sufficient magnitude. In order to be laser proof *a tube must be made entirely of metal*. All laser tubes have a large external diameter relatively to internal diameter and a number of tubes have been used (Table 7.7 and Figure 7.14).

Microlaryngoscopy tubes

These have a small internal and external diameter and are designed specifically for endoscopy procedures of the larynx. A common size is 5.0 mm but both the length and cuff size are appropriate for use in adults (Figure 7.15). They are soft and atraumatic and particularly useful for benign vocal cord

Table 7.7 Laser tubes

Laser tube	Properties
Norton (Oswald-Norton)	Made entirely of steel and therefore laser proof Reusable Flexible with a spiral wound stainless steel wall, no cuff and a relatively large, rough, external diameter Wet packs used to provide a seal for intermittent positive pressure ventilation (IPPV)
Sheridan Laser-track	Red rubber Single use Spiral wrapped with embossed copper foil from the cuff to proximal end of tube* Embossing disperses beam Outer fabric covering is soaked with water prior to use
Mallinckrodt Laser Flex	Corrugated stainless steel shaft Single use Two cuffs in case of intra-operative perforation* cuff may be foam filled
Xomed Laser – shield II	Silicone tube wrapped in aluminium foil and overwrapped with Teflon tape Smooth atraumatic exterior Methylene blue crystals in the cuff allow early detection of perforation*
Bivona	Metallic core Single use Silicone covering Foam filled cuff High incidence of sore throat

*Cuff inflation is with saline.

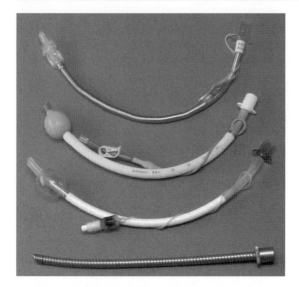

Figure 7.14 Laser tubes: from bottom Norton, Xomed, Sheridan, Mallinckrodt.

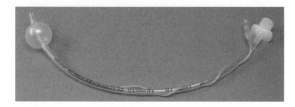

Figure 7.15 Microlaryngeal tube.

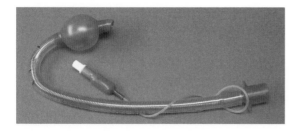

Figure 7.16 Laryngectomy tube.

lesions where placement is undertaken in a controlled, precise manner with no injury to the glottis. As they warm to body temperature, they soften and may kink at the point at which they emerge from the mouth or nose.

Laryngectomy (Montandon) tube

This is J-shaped (Figure 7.16) for insertion into the distal trachea following laryngectomy and

Symbols Key

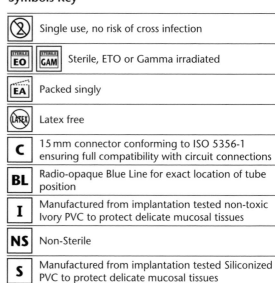

Ⓧ	Single use, no risk of cross infection
STERILE EO / STERILE GAM	Sterile, ETO or Gamma irradiated
EA	Packed singly
LATEX	Latex free
C	15 mm connector conforming to ISO 5356-1 ensuring full compatibility with circuit connections
BL	Radio-opaque Blue Line for exact location of tube position
I	Manufactured from implantation tested non-toxic Ivory PVC to protect delicate mucosal tissues
NS	Non-Sterile
S	Manufactured from implantation tested Siliconized PVC to protect delicate mucosal tissues
10	Packed quantity

Figure 7.17 Meaning of symbols found on tube or packaging.

allows the breathing circuit to be connected at some distance from the stoma. In some versions the cuff is sited at the end of the tube and there is no distal bevel at all to prevent accidental endobronchial intubation.

Key points

- Tube size is internal diameter in millimetres.
- Narrow (small) tubes are easier to insert and cause less morbidity.
- High volume, low pressure cuffs are inherently safer than low volume, high pressure cuffs.
- Intracuff pressure always equals or exceeds lateral wall pressure.
- If lateral wall pressure exceeds mucosal perfusion pressure ischaemia results.
- Safe lateral wall pressure is 20–30 cmH$_2$O.
- Monitoring intracuff pressure is recommended.
- Cuff inflation with air results in an increase in pressure during nitrous oxide anaesthesia.
- Cuff inflation with inspired gas mixture results in a decrease in cuff pressure.

- Saline provides stable cuff pressures but is more difficult to use.
- Consider fire triangle when using tracheal tube for laser surgery.

Further reading

Bolder PM, Healy TE, Bolder AR, Beatty PC, Kay B. The extra work of breathing through adult endotracheal tubes. *Anesth Anal* 1986; **65**: 853–859.

Crawley BE, Cross DE. Tracheal cuffs: a review and dynamic pressure study. *Anaesthesia* 1975; **30**: 4–11.

Hannallah MS, Sudyerhoud JP. Endotracheal tubes and respiratory care. In: Benumof JL (Ed.). *Airway Management Principles and Practice*. St Louis: Mosby, 1996.

Loesler EA, Hodges M, Gliedman J, Stanley TH, Johansen RK, Yonetani D. Tracheal pathology following short-term intubation with low- and high-pressure endotracheal tube cuffs. *Anesth Anal* 1978; **57**: 577–579.

Mitchell V, Adams T, Calder I. Choice of cuff inflation media during nitrous oxide anaesthesia. *Anaesthesia* 1999; **54**: 32–36.

Seegobin RD, Van Hasselt GL. Aspiration beyond endotracheal cuffs. *Can J Anaesth* 1986; **33**: 273.

Shapiro M, Wilson RK, Casar G, Bloom K, Teague RB. Work of breathing through different sized endotracheal tubes. *Crit Care Med* 1986; **14**: 1028–1031.

Tonnesen AS, Vereen AS, Arens JF. Endotracheal tube cuff residual volume and lateral wall pressure in a model trachea. *Anesthesiology* 1981; **55**: 680–683.

Standards Governing endotracheal tubes:

BS (British Standards)
EN (European Standards)
ISO (International Organization for Standards)

CE Council Directive 93/94/EEC 14 June 1993 concerning medical devices:

BS 3487-4	1998	Tracheal Tubes – Part 4: Specification for the Cole Type
BS EN 1782	1998	Tracheal Tubes and Connectors
ISO 5631	1999	Tracheal Tubes and Connectors
ISO 5631-4	1999	Tracheal Tubes – Part 4: Cole Type
BS ISO 14408	1998	Tracheal Tubes Designed for Laser Surgery.

TRACHEAL INTUBATION OF THE ADULT PATIENT 8

J. Henderson

Tracheal intubation is an essential skill in the care of the unconscious, anaesthetized or critically ill patient. Tracheal intubation can be difficult and may result in complications, the most serious being hypoxaemic brain damage and death. Soft tissue damage, sometimes fatal, can be caused by traumatic attempts at intubation. Maintenance of oxygenation must take precedence over all other considerations when difficulty with intubation is experienced and intubation attempts should be deferred until oxygenation is restored.

No technique of airway management is always successful. It is important to have a pre-formulated strategy to cope with unanticipated difficulties. Use of the Difficult Airway Society guidelines is recommended. Many alternative techniques can facilitate tracheal intubation under vision in patients in whom this is not possible with the standard Macintosh laryngoscope. Expertise in at least one alternative visual technique should be acquired and skills maintained; the necessary equipment should be available. Two types of rigid direct laryngoscope (Macintosh and straight) and one indirect rigid laryngoscope (Bullard) will be discussed in this chapter.

Anatomical basis of direct laryngoscopy for tracheal intubation

Successful direct laryngoscopy depends on achieving a line of sight (LOS) (Figure 8.1) from the maxillary teeth to the larynx; management of the base of the tongue and the epiglottis is particularly important (Figure 8.2). The best initial patient position is the 'sniff' position, achieved by flexion of the lower neck and extension of the head. Maximum head extension,

which rotates the maxillary teeth out of the LOS, is probably the most important factor. Changes in position should be made as required to optimize the view. In particular, elevation of the shoulders of obese patients may facilitate head extension.

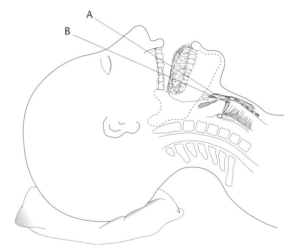

Figure 8.1 LOS with Macintosh (A) and straight (B) laryngoscope. Drawing is based on published scans of patients in the 'sniff' position. The tongue and epiglottis are the principle soft tissue obstructions to the LOS.

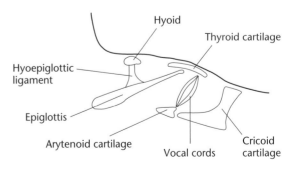

Figure 8.2 Epiglottis and laryngeal cartilages.

The rigid laryngoscope is then used to displace soft tissues out of the LOS. The tongue is displaced horizontally from the LOS, the mandible and hyoid are moved anteriorly, and the epiglottis is elevated (Figure 8.3). A significant lifting force, causing considerable tissue distortion, may be required in direct laryngoscopy. The vector (magnitude and direction) of this force is adjusted to achieve the optimum view of the larynx. The maximum force is applied close to the epiglottis and the direction is at right angles to the LOS. Some factors which can impair achievement of a LOS and may cause difficulties with direct laryngoscopy are shown in Table 8.1. Pre-operative airway assessment is performed with the aim of predicting the probability of failure to achieve a LOS as a consequence of adverse anatomical or pathological factors. Some conditions such as lingual tonsil hyperplasia cannot be detected at pre-anaesthetic assessment.

Preparation

If, following history and examination of the patient, no difficulties are anticipated with airway management, preparations are made for tracheal intubation under general anaesthesia. Adequate personnel, drugs and equipment must be available. A minimum list of equipment is shown in Table 8.2.

Intravenous access is secured and basic monitoring (electrocardiogram (ECG), non-invasive blood pressure (NIBP) and pulse oximeter with beep volume turned on) is established. The patient is pre-oxygenated, and intravenous anaesthesia and neuromuscular block are induced. Paralysis facilitates direct laryngoscopy so that a high success rate can be achieved with minimal trauma. Muscle relaxants must *not* be given if difficulties are anticipated (awake flexible fibreoptic intubation is the technique of choice).

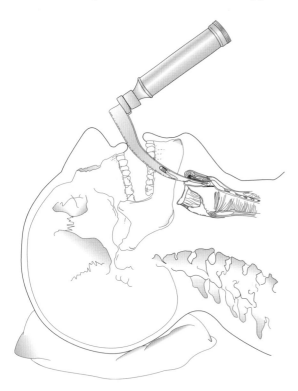

Figure 8.3 Macintosh laryngoscope in optimum position. Maximum mouth opening has been achieved by rotation and advancement of the mandible at the temporo-mandibular joint. The tongue has been displaced to the left of the laryngoscope.

Table 8.1 Some causes of difficult direct laryngoscopy

- Head extension reduced
- Mouth opening limited
- Hypoplastic mandible
- Large incisors or other awkward dentition
- Macroglossia (relative or absolute)
- Narrow mandible
- Lesions of epiglottis or vallecula
- Lingual tonsil hyperplasia

Table 8.2 Basic essential equipment

- Checked anaesthesia machine (or oxygen source and self-inflating resuscitator)
- Range of anaesthesia masks, LMAs oropharyngeal and nasopharyngeal airways
- Two checked laryngoscope handles
- Range of laryngoscope blades (Macintosh and straight)
- Range of tracheal tubes
- Stylet and introducer
- Syringe for cuff inflation
- Lubricant jelly
- Suction apparatus
- Magill forceps
- Tape to secure tube
- Capnograph

Tracheal intubation may also be performed in the patient breathing spontaneously after inhalational induction of anaesthesia. A deep level of inhalational anaesthesia is required and this may be complicated by hypoventilation, arterial hypotension, dysrhythmias and pulmonary aspiration. The conditions created for direct laryngoscopy may be inferior to those achieved with muscle relaxation. Airway patency may be lost when inhalational induction is used in patients presenting with incomplete airway obstruction and rapid creation of a surgical airway may be necessary.

Macintosh laryngoscope and technique of laryngoscopy

The Macintosh technique of laryngoscopy depends on indirect elevation of the epiglottis and it is the most frequently used laryngoscopy technique in most centres. A view of the larynx may be obtained in most patients with this technique.

The patient is positioned with neck flexion and anaesthesia is induced. Once paralysis has been achieved, full head extension completes the positioning manoeuvres and partially opens the patient's mouth. The correct position is often referred to as the 'sniffing' position. This concept was first described by Ivan Magill, who later suggested *draining a pint of beer* as a more memorable description. How much neck flexion should be applied has not been ascertained. Adnet *et al.* compared a 'sniffing' position with simple neck extension and found no benefit in easy to laryngoscope patients. However, they used a pillow of only 7 cm thickness for their sniff position. Horton *et al.* found that most experienced anaesthetists used 29° of flexion of the neck. The Macintosh laryngoscope (size 4 recommended for adult patients) is inserted from right side of mouth to the right of the tongue and advanced carefully, avoiding contact with the mucosa of the palatoglossal arch. As it is advanced, the blade is moved leftwards into the midline to displace the tongue to the left. After ensuring that the lips are not trapped between the laryngoscope blade and the patient's teeth, a lifting force is applied to the laryngoscope handle (in the direction of the handle) to achieve maximum mouth opening as the laryngoscope is further advanced. As the epiglottis comes into view, the tip of the laryngoscope is advanced into the vallecula and the epiglottis is elevated to reveal the laryngeal inlet. The depth of insertion (Figure 8.4) and the lifting force are optimized to achieve the best view of the larynx (Figure 8.5). A considerable lifting force may be necessary (insufficient force is one cause of failure to expose the larynx). Do *not* lever on the teeth as this action risks dental injury and degrades the view of the larynx; the distal

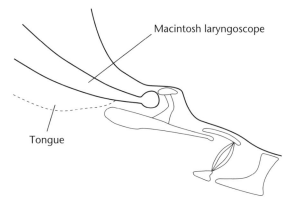

Figure 8.4 Position of epiglottis, tongue and laryngeal cartilages when optimum positioning of the tip of the Macintosh laryngoscope in the vallecula is achieved. The tongue lies entirely to the left of the laryngoscope. Tenting of the hyoepiglottic ligament results in complete elevation of the epiglottis.

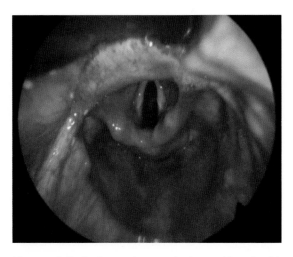

Figure 8.5 Optimum laryngeal view achieved with the Macintosh laryngoscope. In this figure the epiglottis has been allowed to drop a little posteriorly to show the laryngoscope in position in the vallecula.

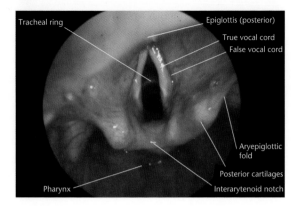

Figure 8.6 Laryngeal anatomy demonstrated with the Macintosh laryngoscope.

Table 8.3 Optimization of view at direct laryngoscopy

- Maximum head extension
- Tongue entirely to the left of the laryngoscope
- Maximum mouth opening
- Optimum depth of laryngoscope insertion
- Maximum lifting force applied in the correct direction
- ELM – applied with anaesthetist's own right hand
- Lift occiput with right hand
- Mandibular protrusion by assistant

anatomy is pushed anteriorly out of the LOS and the proximal blade is rotated into the LOS.

When a good view of the larynx is achieved, the vocal cords, the aryepiglottic folds and posterior cartilages can be identified (Figure 8.6). In other cases, only the posterior cartilages or the epiglottis may be seen. In the worst scenario, only the palate or posterior pharyngeal wall is seen. Occasionally the oesophagus is seen; it is round and puckered, and has no distinctive structures.

If only a poor view of the larynx is achieved, there are three manoeuvres to consider:

1 External laryngeal manipulation (ELM) is applied, usually to the thyroid cartilage, with the anaesthetist's right hand and is adjusted to optimize the view. ELM is different from cricoid pressure, and is an important and integral component of direct laryngoscopy. An assistant is then guided to apply the same ELM.
2 Raising the patient's occiput from the pillow with the right hand, while altering the direction of traction with the laryngoscope to make the axis horizontal or slightly below.
3 Ask an assistant to protrude the mandible by upward pressure on the mandibular rami. Whether this helps in difficult cases is not yet known, but it certainly helps inexperienced laryngoscopists to obtain a view.

If the view remains poor, check that you have used all the manoeuvres in Table 8.3. If a satisfactory view

cannot be achieved, consider blind use of an introducer (next section), a different laryngoscopy technique or abandon laryngoscopy *and* call for the best available help.

When the view of the larynx has been optimized, an assistant retracts the corner of the mouth laterally and the tracheal tube is passed. Do *not* take your eye off the larynx until the tracheal tube has passed into the trachea. Passage of the tube from the right of the LOS (via the corner of the mouth) allows the anaesthetist to observe progress of the tracheal tube towards and through the laryngeal inlet. The optimum shape of the tracheal tube for passage with the Macintosh laryngoscope is that of an ice-hockey stick. A lubricated stylet can help to produce this shape, and it is good practice to have it in position before induction of anaesthesia. Once the tube has entered the trachea, the stylet is removed by an assistant, keeping the tube in place. The tube is passed until the cuff is 2–3 cm beyond the vocal cords, often indicated by a line on the tube. The cuff is then inflated to a just-seal pressure and tracheal position is confirmed. It must be said that some authorities disapprove of the use of stylets. It has been suggested that perforation of the trachea or pharynx is more likely when a stylet is in place.

Confirmation of tube position is *mandatory* as avoidable deaths from hypoxaemia as a consequence of delay or failure to recognize oesophageal intubation continue to occur. The most reliable method is visual confirmation of tube entry into the trachea, but this is not always possible. If visual confirmation is not possible, maintain a high degree of suspicion that the tube might be misplaced and use

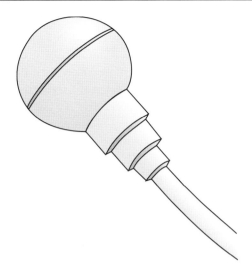

Figure 8.7 The self-inflating bulb has rapidly expanded completely after attachment in a compressed state to the tracheal tube. This confirms correct tracheal position of the tube.

other strategies to ensure proper tube position (see Figure 8.7; Chapter 9).

When oesophageal intubation has been excluded, it is necessary to confirm that the tip of the tube lies in the trachea and not the right main bronchus (Figure 8.8). Auscultation for equal breath sounds over both axillae is performed. Hypoxaemia or an increase in airway pressure should trigger a check for correct position of the tracheal tube, as tubes can be displaced during surgery. Once satisfactory tracheal tube position is confirmed, it is secured so that it will neither come out nor advance into the right main bronchus. Adhesive or tie tape may be used. Record the depth marking on the tube at the patient's teeth or lips.

Finally, it is important to record the best view of the larynx achieved. This information may be vital in planning safe airway management on a subsequent occasion. The standard description is that of Cormack and Lehane (1984): Grade 1 (most of the larynx visible), Grade 2 (posterior structures of the larynx visible), Grade 3 (only the epiglottis visible) and Grade 4 (no laryngeal structure seen).

Success with the Macintosh technique depends on moving the tongue to the left of the laryngoscope and positioning the laryngoscope tip in the vallecula.

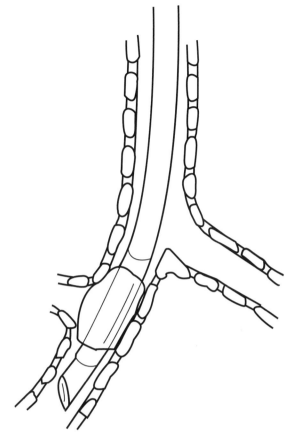

Figure 8.8 Tracheal tube in right main bronchus with cuff occluding right upper lobe bronchus. Only the right middle and lower lobes will be ventilated so that airway pressures will be high and the patient will rapidly become hypoxaemic. There is a risk of barotrauma and the unventilated lung tissue will collapse.

When this laryngoscope position cannot be achieved (Figure 8.9), it is impossible to elevate the epiglottis and to obtain a view of the larynx. The terms 'anterior larynx' and 'floppy epiglottis' are sometimes used erroneously in this situation. These terms impair analysis of the true problems and their use should be abandoned.

There are two important variations on the Macintosh laryngoscope (Figure 8.10). The McCoy laryngoscope uses a lever to flex the tip of the laryngoscope blade. It can improve the view of some Grade 2–3 patients. The left-entry Macintosh laryngoscope is designed for insertion into the left of the mouth. It can be extremely useful in patients with missing upper left maxillary teeth.

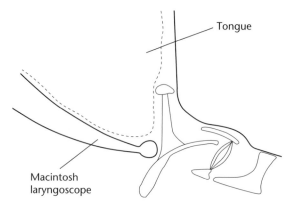

Figure 8.9 Epiglottis, tongue and laryngeal cartilages when the tip of the Macintosh laryngoscope cannot be positioned in the vallecula. It has not proved possible to displace the base of the tongue to the left of the laryngoscope so that it is trapped between the laryngoscope and the hyoid. The epiglottis is not elevated, but is displaced into the LOS. This situation is sometimes erroneously described as 'anterior larynx' or 'floppy epiglottis'.

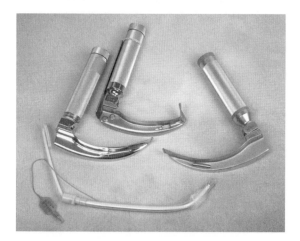

Figure 8.10 Laryngoscopes used with Macintosh technique. Left to right are: Standard Macintosh (size 4), McCoy with tip elevated and left-entry Macintosh. The styleted tracheal tube has been preformed in the shape of an ice-hockey stick. The stylet must be plastic coated and must not protrude beyond the tip of the tracheal tube. This shape can help to guide the tip of the tube to the larynx. Use of a stylet when the larynx is not seen may be more traumatic and less reliable than use of an introducer such as the Eschmann, and is not recommended.

Tracheal tube introducer ('gum-elastic bougie')

A tracheal tube introducer is particularly useful when the laryngeal view is Grade 3 but the epiglottis

can be elevated from the posterior pharyngeal wall. The technique should be practised in supervised simulated difficult tracheal intubation early in anaesthesia training. The most widely used device is the original reusable Eschmann tracheal tube introducer. Other introducers have not been studied as fully, and the incidence of complications may be higher with stiffer devices.

The Macintosh laryngoscope is introduced as described above and the view is optimized and maintained. The larynx should lie in the midline behind the epiglottis. The introducer is curved so that it will pass behind the epiglottis and then come anteriorly to pass between the vocal cords. It is passed gently from a position lateral to the midline. The most useful signs of passage into the trachea are a sensation of clicks as the introducer hits the tracheal cartilages, and increased resistance to passage ('hold-up') when the tip reaches the carina; these signs should always be sought. The tracheal tube is then passed over the introducer ('railroaded') into the trachea (Figure 8.11). The laryngoscope position is maintained to create the most direct route, and the tube is rotated 90° anticlockwise (bevel down) during the passage. Use of a narrow tracheal tube facilitates railroading. Use of all blind techniques should be limited to a few gentle attempts.

Straight laryngoscope (paraglossal technique)

Direct laryngoscopy with the straight laryngoscope (Figure 8.12) was the first technique (Elsberg, 1910) to allow tracheal intubation under vision. It can facilitate tracheal intubation under vision in most patients in whom this proves impossible with the Macintosh laryngoscope. Factors which contribute to the better view achieved with the straight laryngoscope are more effective displacement of the tongue from the LOS and more reliable elevation of the epiglottis (Figure 8.13). The straight laryngoscope may have particular niche roles in patients with lesions in the region of the vallecula or epiglottis, and in patients with a gap in the right upper

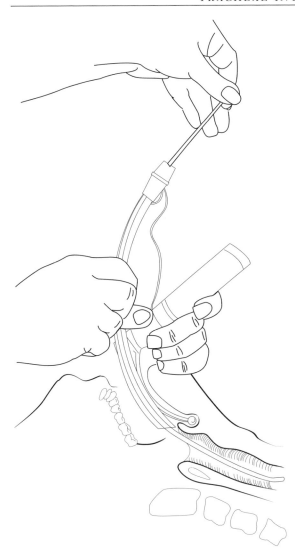

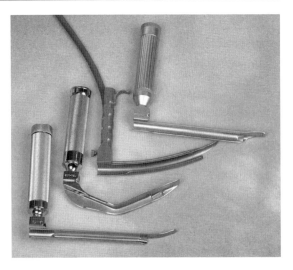

Figure 8.12 Laryngoscopes used with paraglossal straight laryngoscopy technique. Left to right: Miller, Belscope, Piquet-Crinquette-Vilette (PCV) and Henderson. Although the PCV has a gentle curve, it is possible to obtain a LOS through the lumen. The PCV and Henderson have a semi-tubular cross-section to facilitate passage of the tracheal tube.

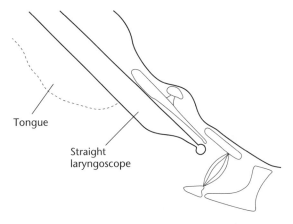

Tongue

Straight
laryngoscope

Figure 8.11 Passage ('railroading') of a tracheal tube over an introducer. The Macintosh laryngoscope has been kept in the optimum position. The assistant holds the proximal end of the introducer while the anaesthetist advances the tube. Reproduced with permission from Figure 13.3.5(b) in Management des schwierigen Atemwegs, ed Dörges und Paschen, published in 2004 by Springer Verlag.

Figure 8.13 Management of tongue, epiglottis and laryngeal cartilages with the straight laryngoscope. In comparison with the Macintosh laryngoscope, tongue control is better and elevation of the epiglottis more reliable.

dentition (Figure 8.14). The technique is different from the Macintosh technique, and effort and commitment are required for its mastery. Differences from the Macintosh technique will be highlighted.

Maximum head extension facilitates insertion of the laryngoscope and ensures minimal contact with the maxillary teeth. Leftward rotation of the patient's

head can be useful. The laryngoscope is inserted to the right of the midline and passed along the paraglossal gutter to the right side of the tongue. Maximum mouth opening may require deliberate attention and the scissor technique (right thumb pressing on the mandibular teeth, index or middle finger pressing on the maxillary teeth) can be useful. When difficulty is experienced, the proximal

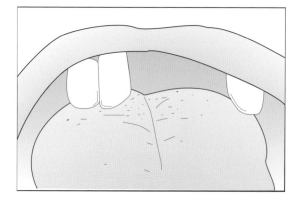

Figure 8.14 Dental pattern associated with difficulty with the Macintosh laryngoscope. Passage of the straight laryngoscope through the upper right gap in dentition is usually straightforward and effective.

end of the laryngoscope should be positioned as far lateral in the mouth as possible (erroneously described as the 'retromolar' technique). The tip of the laryngoscope is passed posterior to the epiglottis and sufficient lifting force is applied to achieve maximum elevation of the epiglottis (Figure 8.15). The tip should finish close to the anterior commissure of the larynx (Figure 8.16), so that an inadvertent backward movement of the laryngoscope will not result in loss of control of the epiglottis. This position can also facilitate passage of the tracheal tube. If the vocal cords are not seen, it is likely that the laryngoscope tip is in the right pyriform fossa, and leftward rotation of the tip will move it into the midline, posterior to the epiglottis. If the tip lies in the oesophagus (deliberate passage into the oesophagus is not recommended), it will be posterior to the cricoid cartilage and ELM reveals a unique sensation of rolling the larynx on the tip of the blade. If the view remains poor after the tip is properly positioned, use of the manoeuvres (Table 8.3) described with the Macintosh is recommended.

The tracheal tube is passed when the optimum view of the larynx has been achieved. If an incomplete view of the larynx is achieved, an introducer should be passed into the trachea under vision, with subsequent railroading of the tube. Blind passage of an introducer is not recommended with the paraglossal straight laryngoscopy technique. Verification of the tracheal tube position (Figure 8.17), cuff inflation

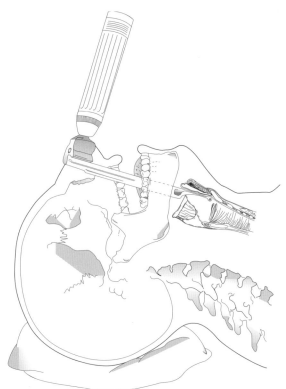

Figure 8.15 Straight laryngoscope in optimum position. The laryngoscope is positioned in the right side of the mouth. Maximum mouth opening has been achieved by rotation and advancement of the mandible at the temporo-mandibular joint. The tongue has been displaced to the left of the laryngoscope. The tip of the laryngoscope is posterior to the epiglottis and close to the anterior commissure of the vocal cords.

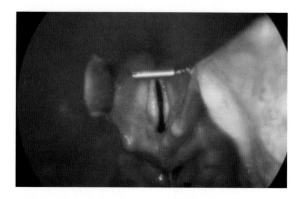

Figure 8.16 View achieved with the straight laryngoscope. The tip is posterior to the epiglottis and close to the anterior commissure. In some patients the right aryepiglottic fold overlies the right vocal cord to some extent when the laryngoscope is passed from the side of the mouth.

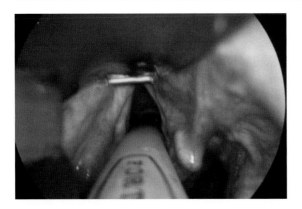

Figure 8.17 Visual confirmation of tracheal intubation with the straight laryngoscope.

and securing the tube are identical to the Macintosh technique.

Bullard-type laryngoscope

The Bullard laryngoscope was introduced in the late 1980s. It is an anatomically shaped rigid fibre-optic laryngoscope, which allows vision of the larynx without the need for significant distortion of tissues. The larynx can be seen in patients in whom this proves difficult or impossible with conventional direct laryngoscopy. This view can be achieved while the patient's head is in a neutral position (Figure 8.18). The Bullard laryngoscope is relatively simple and can be used easily in a ward or emergency room environment. It may also be used in the awake patient under topical anaesthesia. Optimal use requires regular practice.

Intubating laryngeal mask airway

The original laryngeal mask airway (LMA™ Classic) was not designed as a conduit for tracheal intubation, and blind intubation through this device has a low success rate. Use of an Aintree catheter over a flexible fibreoptic laryngoscope can facilitate tracheal intubation through an LMA™ Classic. The intubating LMA (ILMA™) was designed as a conduit for tracheal intubation. Tracheal intubation may be achieved either blindly or under vision (Figure 8.19)

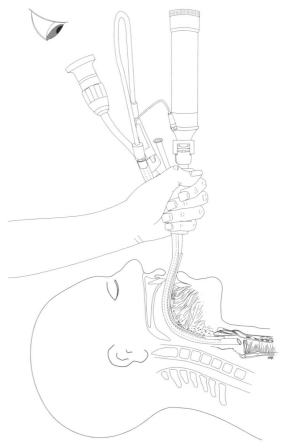

Figure 8.18 Tracheal intubation with the Bullard laryngoscope. The laryngoscope is in the midline and the tip lies posterior to the epiglottis. The head is in a neutral position. The mandible has not been advanced – minimal lifting force is required with this laryngoscope. The tip of the laryngoscope lies posterior to the epiglottis and the tracheal tube has been advanced off the stylet towards the trachea.

(recommended) achieved with a flexible fibreoptic laryngoscope. A high success rate is possible. The recommended technique differs in many respects from the LMA™ Classic, so that users should study the manufacturer's educational material and use the technique during elective surgery.

Other techniques

Macewen (1880) first used his fingers (digital technique) to guide the tracheal tube to the larynx and this technique may still be useful on its own or as

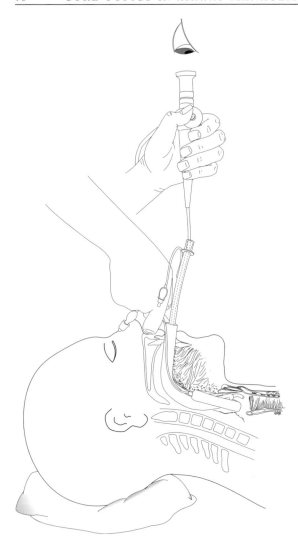

Figure 8.19 Fibreoptic intubation through the ILMA™. The epiglottis is elevated by the epiglottic elevator bar of the device. The tip of the fibrescope is then advanced into the trachea under vision and the tracheal tube is subsequently railroaded over it.

part of composite techniques. A variety of other combined techniques have been described and they can be useful in some situations.

Nasotracheal intubation

Nasotracheal intubation is necessary when the oral route is not available. The nasal route should be used in patients with a history (old or new) of basal skull fracture *only* if there is no alternative. A history of trans-sphenoidal pituitary surgery is also a contraindication to blind passage of a nasal tube.

The risk of damage to nasal polyps and turbinates can be reduced by passage through the nasal cavity under vision (flexible fibreoptic laryngoscope), but traditional techniques of nasotracheal intubation are still widely used. Whenever possible, the nasal mucosa should be shrunk with a vasoconstrictor before induction of anaesthesia. Nasotracheal intubation is usually performed after administration of intravenous anaesthetic and paralysis of the patient. A long narrow cuffed tube (not larger than 7.5 mm for males and 7.0 mm for females) is warmed before use. It is inserted into the anterior nasal cavity. Passage of a suction catheter through the tracheal tube and the nasopharynx, to be followed by the tracheal tube, can reduce the risk of submucosal passage of the tube. Gentle rotation of a narrower tube or use of the other nasal cavity should be considered if there is resistance to passage. The tube is advanced between the palate and posterior pharyngeal wall, towards the larynx.

A laryngoscope is used to facilitate nasotracheal intubation under vision and it should be positioned once the tube tip has reached the oropharynx. Head extension may be used to bring the tip of the tracheal tube anteriorly. Further advancement of the tracheal tube may be facilitated by head and neck flexion, which aligns the axis of tip of the tube with that of trachea. An alternative technique is to use Magill forceps to grasp the tracheal tube (avoiding the cuff) and guide it into the trachea. An assistant then advances the tube.

Rowbotham and Magill (1921) developed the technique of blind nasal intubation in the patient breathing spontaneously. Deep inhalational anaesthesia was used originally, but the technique can be performed in the awake patient under topical anaesthesia. Advancement of the tracheal tube is guided by changes in breath sounds at the proximal end of the tube (amplification by a whistle can be very helpful) and by palpation of the tissues. Blind nasal intubation may still be useful when flexible fibreoptic laryngoscopy fails or is not available. Blind nasal intubation in the apnoeic patient has a low success rate and its use is not recommended in the patient undergoing elective surgery.

Key points

- Quantify and record an airway assessment for every patient before induction of anaesthesia.
- Do not use muscle relaxants if you suspect any problems with tracheal intubation, mask ventilation or rescue techniques.
- Assemble suitable equipment and personnel before inducing anaesthesia.
- The first attempt at tracheal intubation should be the best.
- Always check and optimize: head extension, mouth opening, tongue control, lifting force and ELM.
- Always optimize the view of the larynx before passing the tracheal tube under vision.
- When the introducer is used blindly, be gentle in order to minimize the risk of trauma and to facilitate verification of tracheal position. No more than three attempts should be made.
- Develop a good range of airway skills. The Macintosh laryngoscope, introducer and laryngeal mask are not enough for every patient.
- The straight and Bullard laryngoscopes offer unique advantages and there is good evidence of their value. They should be used regularly.
- Nasotracheal intubation may cause trauma. It should be performed gently, ideally under fibreoptic control.

Further reading

Adnet F, Baillard C, Borron SW *et al*. Randomized study comparing the 'sniffing position' with simple head extension for laryngoscopic view in elective surgery patients. *Anesthesiology* 2001; **95**: 836–841.

American Society of Anesthesiologists Task Force on Management of the Difficult Airway. Practice guidelines for management of the difficult airway. An updated report by the American Society of Anesthesiologists Task Force on Management of the Difficult Airway. *Anesthesiology* 2003; **98**: 1269–1277.

Benumof JL. Conventional (laryngoscopic) orotracheal and nasotracheal intubation (single-lumen tube). In: Benumof JL (Ed.). *Airway Management*. St. Louis: Mosby-Year Book, 1996; pp. 261–276.

Burkle CM, Zepeda FA, Bacon DR, Rose SH. A historical perspective on the use of the laryngoscope as a tool in anesthesiology. *Anesthesiology* 2004; **100**: 1003–1006.

Crosby ET, Cleland MJ. Bullard laryngoscope: keeping its act together. *Anesth Analg* 1999; **89**: 266.

Crosby ET, Cooper RM, Douglas MJ *et al*. The unanticipated difficult airway with recommendations for management. *Can J Anaesth* 1998; **45**: 757–776.

Domino KB, Posner KL, Caplan RA, Cheney FW. Airway injury during anesthesia: a closed claims analysis. *Anesthesiology* 1999; **91**: 1703–1711.

Henderson JJ. The use of paraglossal straight blade laryngoscopy in difficult tracheal intubation. *Anaesthesia* 1997; **52**: 552–560.

Henderson JJ. Questions about the Macintosh laryngoscope and technique of laryngoscopy. *Eur J Anaesthesiol* 2000; **17**: 2–5.

Henderson JJ, Popat MT, Latto IP, Pearce AC. Difficult Airway Society guidelines for management of the unanticipated difficult intubation. *Anaesthesia* 2004; **59**: 675–694.

Horton WA, Fahy L, Charters P. Defining a standard intubating position using 'angle finder'. *Br J Anaesth* 1989; **62**: 6–12.

Latto P. Management of difficult intubation. In: Latto IP, Vaughan RS (Eds). *Difficulties in Tracheal Intubation*, 2nd edition. London: W.B. Saunders Company Ltd, 1997; pp. 107–160.

Marfin AG, Pandit JJ, Hames KC, Popat M, Yentis SM. Use of the bougie in simulated difficult intubation. 2. Comparison of single-use bougie with multiple-use bougie. *Anaesthesia* 2003; **58**: 852–855.

Schmitt HJ, Mang H. Head and neck elevation beyond the sniffing position improves laryngeal view in cases of difficult direct laryngoscopy. *J Clin Anesth* 2002; **14**: 335–338.

Tamura M, Ishikawa T, Kato R, Isono S, Nishino T. Mandibular advancement improves the laryngeal view during direct laryngoscopy performed by inexperienced physicians. *Anesthesiology* 2004; **100**: 598–601.

The *video tapes* published by AirwayCam (www.airwaycam.com) are a very useful teaching resource.

CONFIRMATION OF TRACHEAL INTUBATION 9

O. Sanehi

Introduction

Misplacement of a tracheal tube is a common complication. The tube may pass into the oesophagus or a main bronchus; this may occur at initial placement or the tube may migrate to one of these positions after movement of the patient. Oesophageal intubation is a preventable complication, which is lethal if unrecognized and which every anaesthetist must remain constantly on guard against.

Reasons for confirming tracheal intubation

The prompt recognition of misplacement is important because of the following:

- If not corrected, oesophageal placement *will* lead to:
  - insufflation of the stomach when attempting to ventilate the lungs (in children this can lead to bradycardia and in all ages it increases the risk of regurgitation of stomach contents);
  - hypoxia, brain damage and/or death.
- If not corrected, bronchial placement may lead to:
  - hypoxaemia from shunting of blood;

  - lung or lobar collapse;
  - increased airway pressure and possible barotrauma/volutrauma.
- Consequently it is vital to:
  - differentiate between a tube which has passed through the vocal cords from one which is in the oesophagus;
  - determine that a tube through the cords is in the trachea and not in a main bronchus.

A variety of tests has been devised to do each of these. The tests reviewed here do not comprise a comprehensive list, but are commonly used, reliable or both. The reliability is evaluated according to estimates of the frequencies of false positives (related to specificity) and negatives (related to sensitivity) (Table 9.1). When reading publications on this topic it is important to be clear as to whether the authors are describing their results in terms of the ability of the test to identify tracheal or oesophageal placement. A 'positive' test might refer to placement in either structure, so that a positive test could indicate that the tube is incorrectly placed (test positive when tube is in oesophagus). In this article a positive result indicates tracheal placement.

Table 9.1 Evaluation of tests

	Actual success (correct tube position)	Actual failure (incorrect tube position)
Test perceives success	True positive	Suggests the tube is correctly placed when it is not (false positive)
Test perceives failure	Suggests the tube is incorrectly placed when it is not (false negative)	True negative

Oesophageal intubation

Methods of differentiating between tracheal and oesophageal intubation

Tests to confirm tracheal (as opposed to oesopha-geal) intubation are listed in Table 9.2.

Since manual ventilation through a tube placed in the oesophagus will insufflate the stomach, methods of detecting such a misplacement *prior to* manual ventilation are of great importance and are separated from those requiring manual ventilation.

Table 9.2 Tests to confirm tracheal (as opposed to oesophageal) intubation

	False positive (suggests the tube is in the trachea when it is in the oesophagus)	False negative (suggests the tube is in the oesophagus when it is in the trachea)
Techniques not requiring manual ventilation *Inspection of the vocal cords* Tracheal intubation is usually performed under direct vision; after placement of the tube, there should be visual confirm-ation that *the tube lies surrounded by the glottic structures*	Infrequent Probably mainly due to displacement of the tube after visualization	None reported If visualization is possible, this is an extremely important test
Palpation of the trachea As a tube passes through the trachea, an assistant palpating the external trachea may *feel vibrations*, likened to rubbing a wash-board, and corresponding to the tube passing the tracheal rings. Such vibrations are absent if the tube passes into the oesophagus	Frequent	Frequent
Oesophageal detector device The oesophageal detector device depends upon applying a negative pressure to the tube immediately after placement. Tracheal place-ment results in *free aspiration of gas* from the lungs; in oesophageal intubation, the walls of the oesophagus collapse around the tube lumen preventing gas flow	Very infrequent An underused test which has the advantages of not being dependent on manual ventilation nor on CO_2 production	Infrequent The few reported examples relate mainly to *delayed*, rather than absent, aspiration of gas, in patients with airway obstruction (e.g. bronchial intubation, bronchospasm)
Techniques requiring manual ventilation *Sounds* The *absence of a characteristic flatus-like sound* produced during manual ventilation suggests that the tube is correctly placed; presence of such a sound suggests oesophageal placement	Anecdotally frequent	Anecdotally frequent
Compliance A *'normal' compliance*, (indicated by how hard the reservoir bag must be squeezed for chest expansion) is elicited if the tube is tracheal	Frequent	Frequent But computer-aided techniques are more reliable
Inspection of the chest *Good expansion of the chest* on manual venti-lation suggests correct placement; poor expansion suggests oesophageal intubation	Frequent	Frequent

	False positive (suggests the tube is in the trachea when it is in the oesophagus)	False negative (suggests the tube is in the oesophagus when it is in the trachea)
Auscultation of the epigastrium Manual ventilation through a tube placed in the trachea *does not produce gurgling* heard on auscultating the epigastrium	None reported If the tube is in the oesophagus, there is almost certain to be gurgling	Infrequent
Auscultation of the chest Breath sounds auscultated at the axillae suggest correct tracheal placement	Frequent	Frequent
CO_2 detection Capnography – *a normal capnogram for at least six breaths* suggests tracheal intubation	Very infrequent CO_2 in the stomach (e.g. fizzy drinks) may cause confusion during the first few breaths but is likely to be washed out by six breaths	Infrequent Examples are cardiac arrest, severe bronchospasm and large gas leaks (in all of which CO_2 is not delivered to the capnograph)
Capnometry – a change in *indicator to denote CO_2* suggests tracheal intubation	Infrequent The lack of a graphic display makes CO_2 in the stomach producing a false positive more of a reality	Infrequent See above
Endoscopy Although fibreoptic bronchoscopy can *visually confirm tracheal placement*, its use when suspecting oesophageal intubation is likely to lead to unacceptable delay	Unacceptable delay	Unacceptable delay

CO_2: carbon dioxide.

Taking corrective action in suspected oesophageal intubation

It is important to take corrective action promptly for reasons discussed above. Rapid confirmation of misplacement by visualization of the tube and the laryngeal opening should be attempted – if this is not possible, the tube should be removed anyway (*if in doubt, take it out*). More recently, passing an additional tube, leaving the suspect one *in situ*, has been advocated.

Bronchial intubation

Methods of differentiating between tracheal and bronchial intubation

Tests to confirm tracheal (as opposed to bronchial) intubation are illustrated in Table 9.3.

Unfortunately, none of the easily used tests are very reliable, and desaturation is often the reason that bronchial intubation is suspected and detected.

Taking corrective action in suspected bronchial intubation

If bronchial intubation is suspected, the tube should be gradually withdrawn and reassessment undertaken.

Developing a routine

As can be seen from the tables, there are no perfect tests and so a variety of techniques is used in every case. A suggested routine, combining tests which have low error rates with those which are easily

Table 9.3 Tests to confirm tracheal (as opposed to bronchial) intubation

	False positive (suggests the tube is in the trachea when it is in a main bronchus)	False negative (suggests the tube is in a main bronchus when it is in the trachea)
Compliance A 'normal' compliance, (indicated by how hard the reservoir bag must be squeezed for chest expansion) is detected if the tube is tracheal, a low compliance if it is bronchial	Frequent	Frequent There are many different causes of decreased chest compliance
Inspection of the chest *Equal expansion of both sides of the chest* on manual ventilation suggests correct tracheal placement	Frequent	Frequent
Auscultation of the chest Breath sounds heard on auscultating *both axillae* lines suggest correct tracheal placement and at only one, bronchial placement	Frequent	Frequent
Endoscopy Fibreoptic bronchoscopic *visualization* of the trachea confirms tracheal intubation	Operator dependent	Operator dependent
Radiography The position of the *tube relative to the carina* may be seen on a chest X-ray	Not reported	Not reported

performed, is as follows:

- visualization of the tube between the vocal cords;
- use of the oesophageal detector device;
- inspection of chest expansion;
- auscultation of the epigastrium and the axillae;
- capnography.

Confirmation in adverse circumstances

Developing a routine which includes some reliable, simple tests can be useful in situations in which more sophisticated tests are not possible. For example, the use of capnography to the exclusion of other tests risks missing oesophageal placement in areas where such a facility is absent – for instance during pre-hospital care, in hospital wards and some accident departments and intensive care units.

Key points

- Misplacement is common, and has potentially disastrous sequelae.

- A correctly positioned tube may migrate to an incorrect position and so a high degree of suspicion is mandatory.
- No single test is 100% reliable and so a routine of a combination of tests should be developed.
- *If in doubt, take it out.*

Further reading

Anderson KH, Hald J. Assessing the position of the tracheal tube. The reliability of different methods. *Anaesthesia* 1989; **44**: 984–985.

Clyburn P, Rosen M. Accidental oesophageal intubation. *Br J Anaesth* 1994; **73**: 55–63.

Falk JL, Rackow EC, Weil MH. End tidal carbon dioxide concentration during cardiopulmonary resuscitation. *New Eng J Med* 1988; **318**: 607–611.

Kasper CL, Deem S. The self-inflating bulb to detect oesophageal intubation during emergency airway management. *Anesthesiology* 1998; **88**: 898–902.

McCoy EP, Russell WJ, Webb RK. Accidental bronchial intubation. An analysis of AIMS incident reports from 1988 to 1994 inclusive. *Anaesthesia* 1997; **52**: 24–31.

Sanehi O, Calder I. Capnography and the differentiation between tracheal and oesophageal intubation. *Anaesthesia* 1999; **54**: 604–605.

Tanigawa K, Takeda T, Goto E, Tanaka K. The efficacy of esophageal detector devices in verifying tracheal tube placement: a randomized cross-over study of out-of-hospital cardiac arrest patients. *Anesth Analg* 2001; **92**: 375–378.

Wee MY. The oesophageal detector device. Assessment of a new method to distinguish oesophageal from tracheal intubation. *Anaesthesia* 1988; **43**: 27–29.

EXTUBATION

10

H. Gray

Introduction

There is a fundamental problem attached to extubation. If the tube is removed when airway reflexes are recovered then the presence of the tube will make the patient uncomfortable and sympathetically stimulated. If the tube is removed before the reflexes have returned, then the patient is at risk of aspiration and loss of airway. The former situation may be safer but aesthetically displeasing, while the latter may be nicer to watch but less safe.

Few (if any) experienced anaesthetists approach extubation with total confidence that their patient will suffer no adverse event and their own dignity will be unruffled. It is also true that nowadays we get much less practice in extubation because the laryngeal mask has drastically reduced the need for intubation.

There have never been, and there are unlikely to be, any randomized controlled trials of extubation methods. Extubation remains the 'Cinderella' of management of the difficult airway. In the UK the *Difficult Airway Society Guidelines* do not include advice on the management of extubation, although similar guidelines from Canada and the USA include some advice. Articles on the management of extubation are few and far between, and by nature are full of opinion and very little in the way of evidence-based medicine. Basic questions, such as does coughing at extubation have any influence on postoperative complications like haematoma formation after neuro-, ENT (ear, nose and throat), plastic or eye surgery are unanswered.

However, anaesthesia providers are increasingly recognizing the importance of the emergence, extubation and recovery period as an important contributor to anaesthetic morbidity, and focusing efforts at improving delivery of a quality service in this area.

Problems with extubation

Extubation is rarely impossible but on at least one occasion a double-lumen tube has had to be surgically excised. Extubation problems account for 7% of all respiratory related injuries in the *American Society of Anesthesiologists (ASA) Closed Claim Project* database. Preventable anaesthetic factors lead to 0.19% of all anaesthetized patients requiring an emergency re-intubation.

In the UK it has been shown that complications occurring immediately after tracheal extubation occur nearly three times as frequently as respiratory problems at induction of anaesthesia (4.6% vs. 12.6%). Coughing, desaturation and airway obstruction are all relatively common. Adverse events are more common after extubation in patients who smoke.

The post-extubation patient is particularly at risk for anaesthetic morbidity from:

- *Laryngospasm*: See later.
- *Aspiration*: One-third of aspiration events occur after extubation.
- *Inadequate airway patency* includes:
  - inadequate reversal of muscle relaxation;
  - oedema/haematomas;
  - lingual/tongue oedema;
  - vocal cord paralysis/dysfunction causing paradoxical adduction of the vocal cords during inspiration.
- *Inadequate ventilatory drive*: Opioids and volatile agents blunt response to hypoxia and alter carbon dioxide (CO_2) response curve.

- *Deranged lung function*: Increase in (dead space) as the endotracheal tube (ETT) is replaced by upper airway volume. Arterial oxygen saturation (SaO_2) is <90% in 20–30% of patients extubated without supplementary O_2.

Extubation has a number of undesirable effects, particularly, if it is associated with 'bucking' (a forceful and protracted cough that mimics a Valsalva manoeuvre).

- Coughing/bucking
  - Causes abrupt rises in intracavity pressures with increased intrathoracic pressure leading to decreased venous return.
  - Bucking causes a decrease in functional residual capacity (FRC) and associated atelectasis.
- Cardiovascular
  - 10–30% increase in blood pressure (BP) and heart rate (HR) lasting 5–15 min associated with 40–50% decreased ejection fraction in patients with coronary artery disease.
- Neurological
  - Suctioning unconscious intensive care unit (ICU) patients causes intracranial pressure (ICP) to rise by 15 mmHg for 3–5 min.
  - Extubation is likely to produce similar effects or worse if intracranial compliance is decreased.
- Endocrine
  - Modest transient rises in adrenaline secretion.

Extubation techniques

Any technique should ideally follow Benumof's principles of being:

- Controlled
- Gradual
- Step by step
- Reversible.

The fundamental question that must always be asked is: 'Is this likely to be a potentially difficult airway to manage post-extubation?' Generally an airway that has been difficult to manage during intubation/ placement of a supra-glottic airway device has the potential to be difficult post-extubation.

However, consideration should be given to the following factors that may interact in very different ways for any one individual patient:

- Anaesthesia
- Surgery
- Pathology
- Patient
- Respiratory pattern.

All patients should have a formulated extubation plan as part of the overall airway management plan and this plan should be communicated to all staff likely to be involved; usually the anaesthetist, operating department practitioner and nurses.

The environment in which the ETT is removed should be the one where the patient can be physiologically monitored, and where emergency equipment and appropriately trained staff with airway management skills are immediately available. In most hospitals this will be the operating theatre with an anaesthetist present. However, other suitable environments may exist. Extubation may occur in the recovery room/post-anaesthesia care unit (PACU), and with suitable training and backup, it is successfully performed by experienced nursing staff in some hospitals in the UK.

Before extubation is contemplated adequate spontaneous ventilation should usually be established. If ultra-short acting anaesthetic agents have been used (e.g. balanced anaesthetic combining desflurane and remifentanil) return of respiration may occur concurrently with return of full consciousness and in this situation extubation may be performed prior to established spontaneous respiration.

Adequate spontaneous ventilation includes return of adequate ventilatory drive, tidal volume, respiratory rate, breathing pattern and oxygenation with adequate reversal of neuromuscular blockade.

Position

There is no consensus on the best position for extubation. The 'left lateral, head-down' position is believed by many to offer a reduced chance of pharyngeal fluids being aspirated, as well as giving the best chance of a naturally clear airway. The position also facilitates easy re-intubation for the usual left-handed laryngoscopy.

However, there is now a tendency for the supine, or even head-up position to be used. This may relate to the use of supra-glottic airway devices or the increasing prevalence of diseases such as obesity and chronic obstructive pulmonary disease.

The choice of extubation position reflects a balance between the risks of vomiting post-extubation, and subsequent inhalation and soiling of the lungs (favouring the lateral/head-down position), and potential respiratory embarrassment and ease of assisting ventilation (favouring the supine/head-up position).

Extubation of the uncomplicated airway

The technique of extubation should include the following:

- Administering 100% O_2 for a few minutes.
- Suction of the oro-pharynx *under direct vision*. The common practice of blind suction is regrettable. Trauma to soft tissue is common. Perforation of pharyngeal mucosa with subsequent mediastinitis has been recorded.
- Insert a bite block or oral airway, particularly, if the extubation is to be performed 'awake' – to prevent biting of the tube (a particular hazard with reinforced tubes, which may not regain patency after a bite).
- Deflate the ETT cuff.
- Apply positive pressure to the breathing system reservoir bag and remove the tube. The patient will next breathe out clearing secretions from the supra-glottic region.
- Suction oral secretions.
- Apply mask with high flow O_2 and continuous positive airway pressure (CPAP) as necessary.
- Confirm airway patency and adequacy of ventilation (auscultation of the neck with a stethoscope is a very useful method of monitoring the adequacy of the airway and ventilation).

Other techniques have been tried in an attempt to 'finesse' the standard extubation technique and may have utility in individual situations but studies are either lacking or of very limited number. These techniques include:

- *Extubation and trailing a suction catheter*: It may reduce micro-aspiration of oro-pharyngeal secretions but at the expense of vacuuming O_2 from lungs and producing hypoxia.
- *Extubation on 90% O_2*: It may reduce absorption atelectasis and post-extubation hypoxia.
- *Deep vs. awake extubation*: See later.
- *Intravenous (i.v.) lignocaine 1–1.5 mg/kg 30–90 s prior to extubation*: It can reduce coughing/cardiovascular system (CVS)/ICP changes via a central effect.
- *ETT lignocaine*: 4% lignocaine instilled above or below the ETT cuff.
- *Pharmacology*: Esmolol, glyceryl trinitrate (GTN) infusion, alfentanil, calcium channel blockers and magnesium have all been tried in an attempt to reduce the physiological impact of extubation.

Deep vs. awake extubation

Studies generally demonstrate less bucking, arterial hypertension and destaturation in patients extubated 'deep', which may be of benefit following certain neurosurgical and ophthalmological procedures and in patients with reactive airways. However, this advantage may be offset by an increased incidence of airway obstruction and micro-aspiration. One large UK study showed that 30% of those extubated 'deep' had respiratory complications, twice the rate of those extubated 'awake'. Other studies have shown that the more conscious the patient is on arrival in the PACU the lower the incidence of respiratory complications. In the USA, a difficult airway, obesity and aspiration risk are seen as the major contraindications to deep extubation.

Post-extubation insertion of a laryngeal mask airway (LMA) has been demonstrated to be a useful technique for airway maintenance in the recovery period with less airway obstruction and coughing, and higher SaO_2 than patients who have manual manoeuvres or oro-pharyngeal airways inserted for airway patency.

The most common technique is to place the LMA and inflate its cuff prior to removal of the ETT to ensure that the LMA sits behind the epiglottis and laryngeal inlet.

To achieve a successful deep extubation the end-tidal sevoflurane concentration needs to be >3%. For this purpose sevoflurane is better than isoflurane, which is better than desflurane. Halothane is probably the best of all, but hardly available in the UK.

Awake extubation need not mean coughing and bucking. With careful timing, minimization of head movement and excessive oro-pharyngeal suctioning are combined with deflation of the ETT cuff, while the patient remains deeply anaesthetized; a patient can usually and successfully regain consciousness with the ETT *in situ*.

Consideration also needs to be given to the appropriate environment for the deeply extubated patient to recover from the anaesthetic. In most hospitals the PACU will be more than satisfactory, but some anaesthetists remain with these patients in theatre until the patient is awake. It is possible that slower detection of respiratory problems may contribute to the high incidence of problems seen in the 'deep' patients in the PACU.

The technique that usually ensures smooth deep extubation is to:

- establish spontaneous ventilation with the ETT in place and an end-tidal sevoflurane of >3% in 90–100% O_2;
- suction the oro-pharynx under direct vision with a laryngoscope;
- place oro-pharyngeal airway or LMA;
- deflate ETT cuff;
- ensure there is no reaction to deflation and breathing continues undisturbed;
- remove ETT in single smooth action;
- perform manual manoeuvres as necessary to maintain airway patency and adequate ventilation on 90–100% O_2.

Any movement of the patient (e.g. theatre table to bed) must be done smoothly and minimizing head movement that is likely to promote coughing.

Laryngospasm

A protective mechanism (mediated by the vagus to prevent foreign material entering the larynx) which occurs when patients are extubated between the extremes of very deep and wide awake. It can also be provoked by surgical stimulation. It is particularly common after ENT surgery.

Mild laryngospasm presents with a degree of stridor, while severe laryngospasm causes complete airway obstruction with loss of stridor. It used to be claimed that the glottis would always relax before the patient dies. It is now clear that this is not true. Laryngospasm can provoke negative pressure pulmonary oedema. Re-intubation and positive pressure ventilation is often required, although some cases can be treated with mask CPAP.

Prevention: The incidence of laryngospasm is reduced, particularly in children, if patients are undisturbed (the 'no-touch technique') while they wake up. The patient should be in the lateral recovery position and the only touch allowed is the oximeter clip. Intravenous Magnesium (15 mg/kg i.v. over 20 min) has also been claimed to reduce the incidence after ENT surgery in children.

Simple measures will usually overcome laryngospasm:

- Application of positive end-expiratory pressure (PEEP)/CPAP with 100% O_2.
- Larson's manoeuvre – jaw thrust with bilateral digital pressure in the posterior part of the temporo-mandibular joint (the 'laryngospasm notch') (Figure 10.1).
- Pharyngeal suction.
- Propofol (0.25 mg/kg) is usually very effective and has much reduced the need for suxamethonium.
- Suxamethonium should always be available. Small doses (10–20 mg) are effective. Suxamethonium has a faster onset time in the laryngeal muscles, compared with vecuronium, rocuronium, mivacurium and rapacuronium. A major advantage of suxamethonium is that it is effective when given intramuscularly.

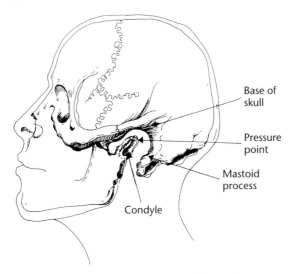

Figure 10.1 The 'laryngospasm notch' bounded anteriorly by the condyle of the mandible, posteriorly by the mastoid process, and superiorly by the base of the skull. Reproduced with permission from Larson (1998).

If laryngospasm is not quickly resolved then it is important to rule out other causes of post-extubation stridor such as:

- soft tissue obstruction;
- throat packs;
- airway oedema (supra- or sub-glottic);
- vocal cord dysfunction;
- external compression (haematoma or obstructed venous drainage);
- aspiration;
- narcotic induced muscle rigidity;
- laryngo- or tracheomalacia.

Extubation of the difficult airway

All remediable factors should be addressed prior to extubation. In particular the temperature should be near normal, fluid balance optimized and whenever possible extubation should be in 'office hours'.

The *ASA Guidelines* recommend the following to be considered:

- the relative merits of awake vs. deep extubation;
- evaluate factors that impact on airway patency/ ventilation;
- formulate a plan for immediate re-intubation;
- the use of a short-term endotracheal ventilation catheter (ETVC) as a conduit/guide for re-intubation.

Most authorities recommend that the anticipated difficult airway is extubated with the patient fully conscious. Undesirable cardiovascular responses can be blunted pharmacologically. If a deep extubation is chosen an LMA may provide a useful means of both maintaining the airway in the waking patient and serving as a conduit for fibre-optically guided re-intubation.

Where peri-glottic swelling is a potential issue, a 'cuff-leak' test can be helpful. Ideally there should be an audible air leak as the cuff of the ETT is deflated confirming adequate airway calibre.

The ETVC

Semi-rigid radio-opaque polyurethane catheters are manufactured by various companies. They are usually 65–85 cm long with outer diameters of 4 mm. They are reasonably rigid to facilitate re-intubation and hollow to facilitate ventilation with removable adaptors allowing passage of the ETT over the catheter. The adaptors can be quickly modified for jet ventilation or attachment to an anaesthetic circuit.

These catheters were originally designed to facilitate safe ETT exchange but experience has demonstrated that they are well tolerated by awake patients even when positioned through the vocal cords in the trachea.

These devices are inserted through the lumen of the ETT and into the trachea prior to extubation and as long as the carina is not stimulated by a too distal placement of the catheter additional analgesia or sedation is not required to ensure patient tolerance.

These catheters can be left in place for as long as 3 days providing a conduit for ETT access to the airway or at least insufflation of O_2.

Extubation failure in the ICU

It is important to separate out the need for an airway from the need for ventilation. Management of failed extubation in the intensive care setting is well documented in the literature. Ventilation failure as a need for re-intubation occurs in up to 20% of intensive care patients at 72 h post-extubation. This failure is associated with increasing age, illness severity, anaemia and duration of ventilation. Objective assessments of cough strength and secretion volume as well physiological measures aimed at assessing respiratory capacity and load aim to reduce this failure rate. The 'Tobin index' is one such measure: $f(\text{rate})/V_t\,(\text{l}) > 100$ has a 95% specificity for predicting extubation failure.

Key points

- Hypoxaemia is commoner at extubation than intubation.
- Always pre-oxygenate before extubation.
- Extubate 'awake' if there is significant risk of aspiration or a difficult airway.
- Consider the use of an ETVC if re-intubation is likely to be difficult.
- Propofol is an effective treatment for laryngospasm, but suxamethonium is effective by the intramuscular route.

Further reading

Asai T, Koga K, Vaughan RS. Respiratory complications associated with tracheal intubation and extubation. *Br J Anaesth* 1998; **80**: 767–775.

Cooper RM. The use of an endotracheal ventilation catheter in the management of difficult extubations. *Can J Anaesth* 1996; **43**: 90–93.

Daley MD, Norman PH, Coveler LA. Tracheal extubation of adult surgical patients while deeply anesthetized: a survey of United States anesthesiologists. *J Clin Anesth* 1999; **11**: 445–452.

Epstein SK. Predicting extubation failure. Is it (on) the cards? *Chest* 2001; **120**: 1061–1063.

Gulhas N, Durmus M, Demirbilek S *et al*. The use of magnesium to prevent laryngospasm after tonsillectomy and adenoidectomy: a preliminary study. *Paediatr Anaesth* 2003; **13**: 43–47.

Inomata S, Yaguchi Y, Taguchi M, Toyooka H. End-tidal concentration for tracheal extubation (MACEX) in adults: comparison with isoflurane. *Br J Anaesth* 1999; **82**: 852–856.

Larson CP. Laryngospasm – the best treatment. *Anesthesiology* 1998; **89**: 1293.

Lien CA, Koff H, Malhotra V, Gadalla F. Emergence and extubation: a systematic approach. *Anesth Analg* 1997; **85**: 1177.

Lim M, Casement J. A review of national difficult airway guidelines. *Roy Coll Anaesth Bulletin* 2004; **24**: 1191–1194.

McConkey PP. Postobstructive pulmonary oedema – a case series and review. *Anaesth Intens Care* 2000; **28**: 72–76.

Miller CG. Management of the difficult intubation in closed malpractice claims. *Am Soc Anesthesiol Newslett* 2000; **64**: 13–16, 19.

Miller KA, Harkin CP, Bailey PL. Postoperative tracheal extubation. *Anesth Analg* 1995; **80**: 149–172.

Probert DJ, Hardman JG. Failed extubation of a double-lumen tube requiring a cricoid split. *Anaesth Intens Care* 2003; **31**: 584–587.

Stix MS, Borromeo CJ, Sciortino GJ, Teague PD. Learning to exchange an endotracheal tube for a laryngeal mask prior to emergence. *Can J Anaesth* 2001; **48**: 795–799.

Tsui BC, Wagner A, Cave D *et al*. The incidence of laryngospasm with a 'no touch' extubation technique after tonsillectomy and adenoidectomy. *Anesth Analg* 2004; **98**: 327–329.

Vaughan RS. Extubation – yesterday and today. *Anaesthesia* 2003; **58**: 949–950.

B. Dercksen & P.A.J. Borg

Light-guided intubation was introduced in 1959 by Yamamura. Since then several intubation devices which use transillumination have been developed. In 1995 Hung introduced the Trachlight, which has proved to be the most popular device. This instrument has been thoroughly evaluated in almost 50 published articles and has been proven to be safe, effective and easy to use in most cases.

Principle of transillumination

The light-guided intubation technique is based on transillumination of the soft tissues of the neck from inside out. A lighted stylet is placed in the endotracheal tube (ET) in such a way that the light source marks the tip of the ET. ET and stylet are introduced into the upper airway and transillumination indicates the position of the tip of the ET in the patient. When transillumination is seen externally at the level of the cricothyroid membrane, the tip of the ET is considered to be distal to the vocal cords, in the larynx. When the ET is further advanced into the trachea, the tip can be followed by means of a moving transilluminated spot.

Instrument

The Trachlight consists of three parts: a handle, a semi-rigid pliable metal stylet and a hollow flexible lightwand (Figure 11.1). The stylet fits inside the hollow lightwand and the ET is mounted over the lightwand. When the stylet is clicked into the active position, the combination of both components plus the ET is semi-rigid but pliable. During the process of intubation the stylet can be retracted out of the

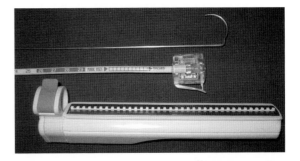

Figure 11.1 The three parts of the Trachlight.

lightwand which turns the lightwand flexible again. This is important because the rigidity facilitates manoeuvring the lightwand through the vocal cords into the larynx, while the flexibility enables safe advancement of the ET further into the trachea.

The tip of the lightwand has a light source which is powered by three AAA batteries in the handle and the on/off switch is located at the back of the handle. The lightwand is connected to the handle by means of sliding rails, which allows adjustment of the lightwand for ETs of differing length. The 15 mm clamp at the distal end of the handle accepts a standard 15 mm ET connector (Figure 11.2).

Intubation technique

The basic oro-tracheal intubation technique will be described below. In the literature several modifications of this technique are described.

Preparation

Stylet and lightwand should be lubricated with silicone spray. The lightwand, with stylet in place, is connected to the handle via the sliding connection. An ET is placed over the lightwand and secured with the 15 mm clamp at the handle. Upward orientation of the bevel, when the ET is advanced into the trachea, will prevent the tip of the ET impacting on the anterior tracheal wall. To position the light source in the tip of the ET, the lightwand is adjusted to the appropriate length with the sliding connection. Then ET, lightwand and stylet are bent in a 90° angle upward at a point indicated on the lightwand (Figure 11.3). Finally the light is checked.

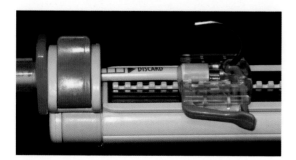

Figure 11.2 Detail of the lightwand and ET connection.

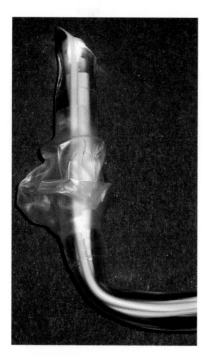

Figure 11.3 The lightwand bend in a 90° upward angle.

Holding and inserting the instrument

The dominant hand holds the instrument in such a way that the on/off switch rests in the palm of that hand, the hook of the stylet fits the ring finger and the thumb rests at the proximal end of the handle (Figure 11.4). With the head in a neutral position the intubator grasps the jaw with one hand, most easily done by putting the thumb in the mouth, and elevates the jaw. After the light has been switched on, the instrument is introduced into the mouth and the lighted tip of the instrument manoeuvred in the direction of the cricothyroid membrane. A bright transilluminated light spot is seen through this membrane when the tip of instrument is below the vocal cords (Figure 11.5). Transillumination at a spot other than the cricothyroid membrane indicates malpositioning. When there is transillumination through the cricothyroid membrane, but less bright than expected, the instrument may have been advanced into the oesophagus. Malposition can be corrected by partly withdrawing the instrument and repositioning it with a gentle 'rocking' movement. In fact the instrument is used to carefully probe the laryngeal entrance. No undue force on tissues can be exerted, as force will bend the instrument and it will not easily damage the patient.

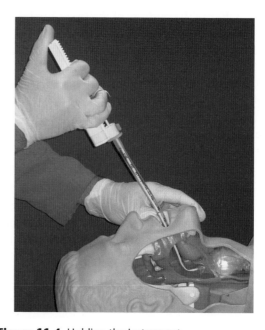

Figure 11.4 Holding the instrument.

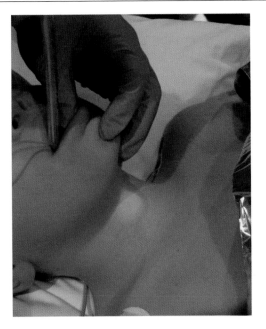

Figure 11.5 Transillumination at cricothyroid membrane.

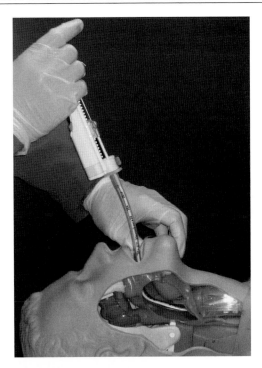

Figure 11.6 Retracting the stylet.

Advancing the tube into the trachea

When one is convinced that the tube has passed the vocal cords, the stylet is retracted. This is done by 'pushing' the instrument deeper into the trachea while preventing the stylet following this movement by holding the ring finger plus stylet in the same position. In this way retraction of the stylet and advancing the ET deeper into the trachea is performed in one single movement (Figure 11.6). The position of the tip of the ET can be traced from outside by following the moving transilluminated spot (Figure 11.7). When the spot is just above the sternal notch, the tip of the ET is halfway between the vocal cords and carina, the cuff of the ET will have passed the vocal cords and so the ET is in the correct position.

Removing the instrument

After releasing the ET from the instrument by unlocking the clamp, the instrument is pulled out. A quick pull is advocated, in order to reduce the friction between ET and lightwand. Reducing this friction aids in preventing dislocation of the ET while retracting the instrument.

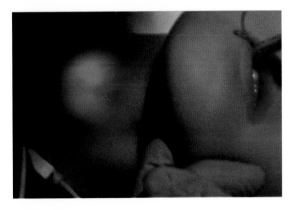

Figure 11.7 Transillumination just above the sternal notch.

Indications and contraindications

The Trachlight is a simple effective 'carried-in-the-pocket' device which has been used for oral intubation in anaesthetized and awake patients. The vectors of force and the route to the larynx are quite unlike direct laryngoscopy. In one study of 950 patients it compared favourably with direct laryngoscopy with a mean intubation time of 16 s, a 92%

success rate for the first intubation attempt and an overall failure rate of 1%. In a subsequent study of 206 patients with a history of, or anticipated, difficult intubation there was a mean intubation time of 26 s and a 1% failure rate. Its chief indication is, then, difficult direct laryngoscopy particularly when there is limited mouth opening, restricted neck movement or difficult dentition. It becomes more difficult to use, or contraindicated, when there is supraglottic or glottic pathology, or when the cricothyroid membrane is not visible due to a short obese neck or an overlying thyroid mass.

Conclusion

Transillumination intubation is a relatively 'blind' technique but the disadvantages of this are balanced by a simple technique which is not difficult to learn, has a high success rate and uses easily portable equipment. Experience should be gained in elective situations before moving to the emergency use.

Key points

- Transillumination (Trachlight) intubation is safe and effective in skilled hands.
- Acquiring skill in elective situations is necessary to be able to apply the technique in emergency situations.
- The Trachlight takes a different route to the same target as the laryngoscope and is, therefore, a useful alternative in case of failed direct laryngoscopy.

- A carefully executed technique with a properly prepared instrument is the key to success.
- Indications for the technique are a known or unexpected difficult airway, or routine use in elective cases.
- In emergency situations there are no specific contraindications to the use of the Trachlight.

Further reading

Agro F, Hung OR, Cataldo R, Carassiti M, Gherardi S. Lightwand intubation using the Trachlight: a brief review of current knowledge. *Can J Anaesth* 2001; **48**: 592–599.

Davis L, Cook-Sather SD, Schreiner MS. Lighted stylet tracheal intubation: a review. *Anesth Analg* 2000; **90**: 745–756.

Graham DH. Lightwand intubation using the Trachlight: a brief review of current knowledge. *Can J Anaesth* 2001; **48**: 1169–1170.

Hung OR, Stewart RD. Lightwand intubation. I. A new lightwand device. *Can J Anaesth* 1995; **42**: 820–825.

Hung OR, Pytka S, Morris I, Murphy M, Launcelott G, Stevens S, MacKay W, Stewart RD. Clinical trial of a new lightwand device (Trachlight) to intubate the trachea. *Anesthesiology* 1995a; **83**: 509–514.

Hung OR, Pytka S, Morris I, Murphy M, Stewart RD. Lightwand intubation. II. Clinical trial of a new lightwand for tracheal intubation in patients with difficult airways. *Can J Anaesth* 1995b; **42**: 826–830.

Lipp M, de Rossi L, Daublander M, Thierbach A. The transillumination technique. An alternative to conventional intubation? *Anaesthesist* 1996; **45**: 923–930.

I. Calder

Dr Peter Murphy (Figure 12.1) was the first to use a flexible endoscope ('scope) to intubate the trachea, while a Registrar at the National Hospital, Queen Square in 1967. He moved to Chicago shortly afterwards, where he still practises.

Flexible fibreoptic intubation is a tremendously useful technique, which every anaesthetist should attempt to master. The advantage of vision, the pre-eminent sense, needs no explanation.

Fibreoptic laryngoscopy is easier in the awake patient. The less experienced you are, the more inclined to an 'awake' procedure you should be.

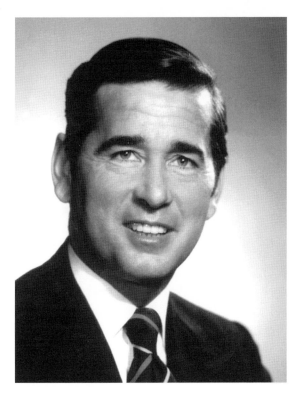

Figure 12.1 Dr Peter Murphy.

Flexible fibreoptic intubation is not a panacea because of the following:

1 It is relatively slow, not suitable for really rapid airway management.
2 Blood and secretions can easily prevent vision.
3 An air space is required, which may be absent when there is soft tissue swelling.
4 It can be impossible to access a glottis displaced from the midline.

Blind techniques have succeeded when flexible fibre-optics have failed.

How to do it

Make sure the equipment is correct

a Use a television (TV) camera and screen if possible (a bigger view and helpful for assistants).
b Adjust the focus and orientation of the camera.
c Use a mains-powered light source if possible, although battery-powered ones are adequate.
d The easiest tracheal tube to pass off a flexible laryngoscope is the silicone intubating laryngeal mask airway (silicone ILMA) tube, followed by the 'Flexium'-reinforced tube (Mallinkrodt). Ordinary tubes can be used but do not pass as easily.
e Wind the pilot tube round the tube and fix (loosely) with tape.
f Use the smallest size of tube you can; 6 mm for women and 7 mm for men is usual. If you must use a bigger tube consider a two-tube technique (i.e. an uncuffed small tube inside the big one).

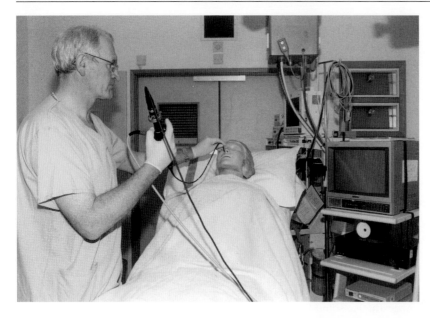

Figure 12.2 The correct position for patient, endoscopist and TV screen.

Get in position

a If possible have the head of the patient raised to 20° or higher.

b Stand by the patient's side. Always use this position, so you are used to it.

c Make sure the TV screen is positioned so you can see it easily.

d A common misconception is that the 'scope needs to be kept straight while out of the body – this is not true and causes unnecessary fatigue; just use both hands when turning the 'scope (Figure 12.2).

Choose a route

a The 'angle of attack' is better with the nasal route, and gagging (and biting) is avoided, but it means a nasal intubation (Figures 12.3 and 12.4).

b The oral route is more difficult in the awake patient – gagging (a glossopharyngeal nerve reflex) is hard to abolish.

Abolish (or attenuate) the airway reflexes

a Approaching the glottis with inadequately obtunded reflexes can cause laryngospasm and total obstruction.

b Topical local anaesthesia needs to be applied in a cautious escalation to avoid glottic irritation and closure.

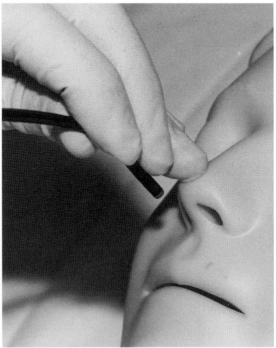

Figure 12.3 The correct angle of approach to the nasal cavity. *Start looking down the endoscope, or at the screen from this point on.*

c Using volatile anaesthetics and spontaneous breathing may be theoretically attractive but fraught with complications in the authors' hands.

d Propofol and remifentanil infusions are more successful.

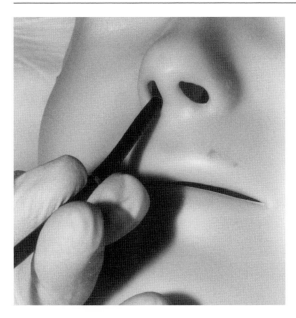

Figure 12.4 Incorrect angle of insertion.

e The best conditions are obtained with muscle relaxants.

f There are occasional 'emergency' situations, for instance where face and neck are rapidly swelling, when the 'scope must be passed and a dose of propofol used to allow passage of the tube.

Clear the airway

a If there are secretions/bleeding use a suction catheter. The suction channel in the 'scope is less effective.

b In the awake patient, asking for a 'deep breath' is very useful.

c For oral intubation the best tongue control is a Duval's forceps, with which the tongue can be very effectively controlled. Jaw thrust and head extension should be applied and occasionally a direct laryngoscope is helpful.

d A variety of oral airways are available, such as the Berman or Ovassapian.

e A dental prop is useful for awake oral fibreoptic intubation, as biting is reliably prevented.

f A trans-tracheal cannula to allow jet ventilation is useful in some patients.

Introduce the endoscope

a Hold the 'scope at the tip and begin looking at the TV screen *before you enter the body*. This ensures correct orientation. Failing to establish orientation is the commonest mistake made by the inexperienced.

b If inexperienced, do not think about which way to rotate the 'scope or move the lever – just try something and do the opposite if it is wrong.

c If you are attempting to endoscope a spontaneously breathing partially obstructed patient, you may find that vision is only possible during *expiration*.

Pass the tube

a Ask an assistant to hold the 'scope.

b Apply lubricating jelly to the distal end of the tube. Run a little saline down the proximal end of the tube, to ease its passage off the 'scope.

c If using a silicone or reinforced tube 'drill' the tube in with many 360° turns keeping *both hands* on the tube at all times (the aim is to get the distal end twisting, which may need several twists at the proximal end until the tube is 'wound up'). Try not to get jelly on your fingers, it destroys your grip.

d If using an ordinary tube you may not be safely able to drill it in and must try less florid twisting (try 180° twists). If the hold up is at glottic level always withdraw before twisting.

e Always check the tube position by auscultation as well as fibreoptically, it is easy to confuse the carina with the divisions of the right main bronchus.

Nasendoscopy

Nasendoscopy is an unfamiliar visual experience for the beginner. The nose has three 'compartments' – the nostrils, the turbinates, and the posterior nasal space. The airway through the three turbinates is multi-channel and each channel is narrow. It is easy to lose orientation. The aim is to identify the septum, inferior turbinate and nasal floor, and establish orientation, *before leaving the*

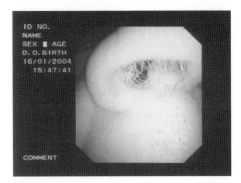

Figure 12.5 Nasendoscopy: Step 1.

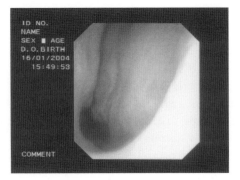

Figure 12.6 Nasendoscopy: Step 2 (Septum on left).

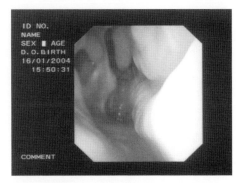

Figure 12.7 Nasendoscopy: Step 3.

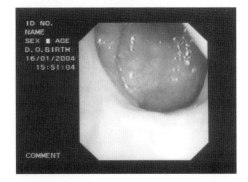

Figure 12.8 Nasendoscopy: Step 4.

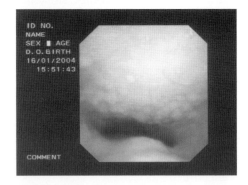

Figure 12.9 Nasendoscopy: Step 5.

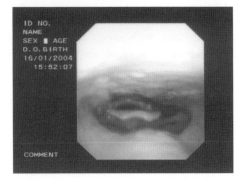

Figure 12.10 Nasendoscopy: Step 6.

nostril. The best route through the turbinates is usually along the floor of the nose. It is very useful to be able to arrive in the posterior nasal space knowing where up and down, left and right are. The route out of the nose is then obvious (which it often is not in unconscious patients):

1 Always start looking at the screen at this point (i.e. check your orientation before entering the nostril). If the airway does not look immediately inviting, have a look in the other side (see Figure 12.5).
2 Identify the septum, floor of nose and inferior turbinate (Figure 12.6).
3 Advance through the turbinate space (Figure 12.7).
4 Enter the posterior nasal space. Soft palate below, nasopharyngeal mucosa ahead (Figure 12.8).
5 Turn down to pass between soft palate and pharyngeal wall (Figure 12.9). This may only be a fissure in the unconscious patient.
6 Identify the epiglottis (Figure 12.10).

Laryngeal mask airway techniques

Little has changed since the first description by Silk. This is both an excellent rescue technique after failed direct laryngoscopy (the laryngeal mask airway (LMA) lifts the glottis out of the blood and secretions that can make fibreoptic vision difficult) and elective procedure where difficulty is expected.

Pass the LMA

A size 3 or 4 will allow a 6 mm Flexilum-reinforced tube (Mallinkrodt) to pass. The Flexilum tubes are 33 cm long. A size 5 LMA will permit passage of a 6.5 or 7 mm Flexilum, but you need to cut 5 cm off the shaft of the LMA to permit enough of the tube to enter the trachea. The shaft of the disposable LMA also needs to be trimmed by the same amount.

If inexperienced, use a catheter mount with a bronchoscopic port to allow preliminary fibreoptic laryngoscopy. Use saline to lubricate the laryngoscope. If the position of the LMA does not give a good view, try adding or removing air from the cuff and/or repositioning it, or getting an assistant to perform jaw thrust.

Pass the endoscope

Stand by the patient's side, because the curve of the endoscope is then a simple one. Advance until the tracheal tube enters the LMA.

Lubricate the tube

Place jelly on the distal 2 in. of the tube and run a little saline between the tube and the 'scope. *Do not let jelly get on your fingers.*

Pass the tube

The tube must be drilled in, with many 360° turns – this is vital, it helps to wind the pilot tube round the tube and loosely tape it in place. This stops the pilot tube flailing round as you 'drill' the tube in. If the LMA needs to be removed or a larger tube needs to be placed, there are two alternatives.

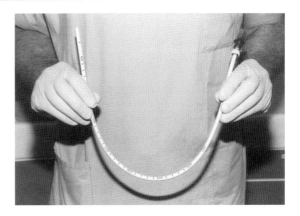

Figure 12.11 The Aintree catheter.

Firstly, the Aintree catheter (Figure 12.11), which is passed over a fibreoptic laryngoscope through the LMA. The LMA is then removed and a tracheal tube passed over the catheter. It is wise to lubricate the inside of the catheter before placing it on the endoscope as it is a snug fit; make sure the catheter will come off easily before passing the 'scope. Secondly, one can pass a tube (a polyvinyl chloride, PVC one will do), then pass a gum elastic bougie through it, remove the LMA and pass a definitive tube.

Alternatively, use the ILMA as a conduit for fibreoptic laryngoscopy.

'Awake' fibreoptic intubation

Complete, absolute, wakefulness is rarely a good idea, particularly where the procedure may need to be repeated.

Nasogastric tubes: If a nasogastric tube is going to be required it is sensible to ask the patient to swallow it before the tracheal intubation. It is embarrassing for you, and hazardous for the patient, if you have difficulty passing a nasogastric tube after the trachea is intubated.

Additional oxygen by nasal catheter or 'prongs', drying of secretions with glycopyrrolate (administered as long before as possible), and an undramatic explanation of events are all helpful. Have the patients semi-sitting, stand by their side and maintain eye contact.

Sedation

Amnesia is sensible. You or a colleague may be in difficulty if the patient declines a repeat procedure. A small dose (1 mg) of midazolam is sufficient. Remifentanil has been used in a 'single-drug' technique. Machata and colleagues compared a 'low-dose' regime (0.75 μg/kg bolus then 0.75 μg/kg/min) and a 'high-dose' (1.5 μg/kg bolus then 1.5 μg/kg/min). All patients had 0.05 mg/kg midazolam. They reported excellent conditions with both regimes and more profound sedation with the higher dose. Propofol and remifentanil in a target-controlled infusion (TCI) technique has been reported as successful, as has the combination of dexmedotomidine and ketamine.

Topical anaesthesia

Drying the mucosa with glycopyrrolate makes topicalization more effective, but also increases absorption. Patients will occasionally become hypotensive after intubation, possibly as a result of lidocaine absorption.

It is useful to shrink the nasal mucosa with a vasoconstrictor such as phenylephrine 0.5%, which is supplied in 5% lidocaine by UK pharmacies. Cocaine is very effective but its undeniable toxicity makes its use hard to justify. Two percent lidocaine jelly is convenient for nasal instillation and gargling. 'Spray as you go' lidocaine 2% or 4% is facilitated by passing an epidural catheter (end cut-off) part way down the suction channel. Five millilitres of lidocaine solution is usually sufficient. Toxicity may occur with doses >9 mg/kg. Lidocaine is irritant to the glottis and stridor is not uncommon if topicalization is too aggressive. Filling the nasal passages with 2% gel and asking the patient to sniff will diminish glottic sensation sufficiently to permit direct application of lidocaine.

Formal nerve blocks are rarely required. Glossopharyngeal blocks are less efficacious than topicalization. Crico-thyroid injection of lidocaine is effective but can induce severe coughing and sometimes laryngospasm.

Retrograde techniques

Blood and tissue swelling may make anterograde vision impossible. The fibrescope can be used as an introducer by passing a wire, introduced through the crico-thyroid membrane up the suction channel.

Alternative vision-guided techniques

Video-laryngoscopes

Devices that incorporate a flexible fibreoptic bundle, such as the Glidescope. The image is displayed on a TV screen. The combination with gum elastic bougie is a powerful one.

Rigid nasendoscope

A rigid nasendoscope with an oblique viewing lens (70°) can be used to obtain a glottic view when direct laryngoscopy is impossible. The endoscope is introduced orally and a gum elastic bougie, or tube manoeuvred into the trachea.

Key points

- Get used to standing alongside the patient.
- Use a TV system.
- The LMA provides a successful conduit.
- Flexo-metallic or ILMA tubes are the easiest to pass.
- A 'drilling' technique is the best for passing the tube.
- Do not get lubricating jelly on your fingers.
- The less experienced you are, the more inclined you should be to use an 'awake' technique.

Further reading

Barker KF, Bolton P, Cole S, Coe PA. Ease of passage during fibreoptic intubation: a comparison of three endotracheal tubes. *Acta Anaesth Scand* 2001; **45**: 624–626.

Biro P, Weiss M, Gerber A, Pasch T. Comparison of a new video-optical intubation stylet versus the conventional malleable stylet in simulated difficult tracheal intubation. *Anaesthesia* 2000; **55**: 886–889.

Calder I, Ovassapian A, Calder N. John Logie Baird – fibreoptic pioneer. *J Roy Soc Med* 2000; **93**: 438–439.

Machata AM, Gonano C, Holzer A *et al.* Awake nasotracheal fiberoptic intubation: patient comfort, intubating conditions, and hemodynamic stability during conscious sedation with remifentanil. *Anesth Analg* 2003; **97**: 904–908.

Maktabi MA, Hoffman H, Funk G, From RP. Laryngeal trauma during awake fiberoptic intubation. *Anesth Analg* 2002; **95**: 1112–1114.

McGuire G, el-Beheiry H. Complete upper airway obstruction during awake fibreoptic intubation in patients with unstable cervical spine fractures. *Can J Anaesth* 1999; **46**: 176–178.

Osborn NA, Jackson AP, Smith JE. The laryngeal mask airway as an aid to training in fibreoptic nasotracheal endoscopy. *Anaesthesia* 1998; **53**: 1080–1083.

Osula S, Stockton P, Abdelaziz MM, Walshaw MJ. Intratracheal cocaine induced myocardial infarction: an unusual complication of fibreoptic bronchoscopy. *Thorax* 2003; **58**: 733–734.

Ovassapian A. *Fiberoptic Endoscopy and the Difficult Airway*, 2nd edition. Philadelphia: Lippincott-Raven, 1996.

Popat M. *Practical Fibreoptic Intubation*. Oxford: Butterworth-Heinemann, 2001.

Ravishankar M, Kundra P, Agrawal K *et al.* Rigid nasendoscope with video camera system for intubation in infants with Pierre–Robin sequence. *Br J Anaesth* 2002; **88**: 728–731.

Scher CS, Gitlin MC. Dexmedetomidine and low-dose ketamine provide adequate sedation for awake fibreoptic intubation. *Can J Anaesth* 2003; **50**: 607–610.

Watson NC, Hokanson M, Maltby JR, Todesco JM. The intubating laryngeal mask airway in failed fibreoptic intubation. *Can J Anaesth* 1999; **46**: 376–378.

RETROGRADE INTUBATION   13

A. Pearce

Retrograde intubation is a misnomer since intubation is undertaken in the normal direction over a guide-passed retrogradely. The first description by Butler and Cirillo was of a catheter passed through a healing tracheostomy, up between the vocal cords and out of the mouth, over which a tracheal tube was railroaded. The first author to describe puncture of the intact cricothyroid membrane (CTM) was Waters (1963), then working in Africa. His method was to use a Tuohy needle to puncture the CTM, feed up 'a yard' of plastic tubing similar to an epidural catheter until it exited the mouth and intubate over the catheter.

A literature search in the mid-1990s revealed about 500 retrograde intubations, about 300 of which were in cadavers. Mean intubation time was about 40 s with a 98% success rate. It is, therefore, a simple, effective technique supported by a reasonable body of published work. There are two variants, namely blind and fibreoptic assisted. For the blind technique a purpose-built kit (Figure 13.1) is available from Cook Critical Care, and this will be used for description of the technique. Developments since the original description of blind retrograde by Waters have focused particularly on the guide. The epidural catheter has been replaced by a guidewire with a J-tip, with a diameter sufficient to pass through a 20-G catheter but enough stiffness to provide support for intubation. Intubation does not occur over the guidewire alone, because the difference in size between the wire and tracheal tube means that the tube tip is highly likely to impinge on the larynx. The wire is made fatter and stiffer by a bougie (or wire-stiffener) slid anterogradely, over which the tracheal tube is railroaded.

The indications for blind retrograde are expected or unanticipated difficult direct laryngoscopy. There are

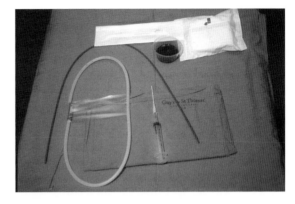

Figure 13.1 Retrograde kit – needle/cannula, wire and wire-stiffener.

Table 13.1 Relative contraindications

Glottic or supraglottic pathology
Bleeding disorder
Infection over CTM
Inaccessible CTM/trachea

now a variety of intubation techniques when direct laryngoscopy is difficult and a blind, invasive procedure is unlikely to be first choice when alternatives such as fibreoptic intubation or the intubating laryngeal mask airway (ILMA) exist. However, in developing countries or difficult circumstances outside hospital where specialized equipment is unavailable, blind retrograde intubation has much to recommend it. The fibreoptic-assisted retrograde technique is useful as a back-up plan when fibreoptic intubation is difficult. Contraindications are listed in Table 13.1.

Blind technique

Intubation may be in the conscious-sedated patient, or in the anaesthetized (usually paralysed) state.

The laryngeal reflexes must be abolished either by topical anaesthesia (3–4 ml 4% lidocaine injection through the CTM or upper trachea), adequate muscle relaxation or deep anaesthesia. The CTM should be identified, the overlying skin cleaned with disinfectant and a sterile drape placed over the body. A right-handed anaesthetist stands on the right side of the patient, stabilizes the larynx with the fingers of the left hand and inserts an ~20-G cannula with syringe attached through the CTM, aspirating continuously. Once the cannula is within the airway, the needle is stabilized, and the cannula slid off and advanced cephalad. There should be no resistance to advancement. The needle is withdrawn and free aspiration of air through the cannula confirmed, to verify that it lies within the airway. Care must be taken in the initial placement of the needle/cannula because the vocal cords are only 1 cm superior to the CTM. The whole length of the cannula is inserted and its tip will be superior to the vocal cords.

The Cook kit contains a J-wire and this is fed up through the cannula. The anaesthetist leaves the wire in the care of an assistant, goes to the top of the table and finds the wire in the pharynx by careful, gentle inspection of the posterior pharyngeal wall using a laryngoscope. The wire is either withdrawn or inserted by the assistant until the anaesthetist can grab the J-tip of the wire with Magill's forceps and carefully withdraw it through the mouth (Figure 13.2). The cannula is left in place so the wire does not act as a cheese-cutter and damage the larynx. The usefulness of the J-tip is that, on appropriate rotation of the wire by the assistant, the J-tip will stand 'proud' of the pharyngeal mucosa and be easier to grasp. Marks indicate when sufficient wire has been withdrawn through the mouth and the cannula is then removed. Care should be taken not to withdraw the wire completely and forceps may be applied to the end protruding externally at the CTM.

The wire-stiffener is placed over the wire, introduced into the oral cavity and advanced until the tip abuts on the internal surface of the CTM. It is on this manoeuvre that success depends and it is possible, particularly with an active glottic closure reflex, for the tip to impact on the larynx rather than pass through the glottic aperture. With correct placement,

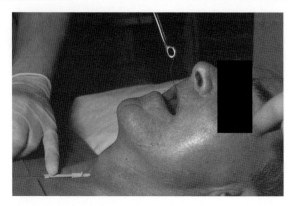

Figure 13.2 Retrograde – withdrawing the wire from the mouth with Magill's forceps.

small repetitive withdrawal/advancements of the wire-stiffener produce a certain feel of engagement and movement of the external wire.

Once the wire-stiffener is in place, it is held firmly while the tracheal tube is placed over it (preferably the smallest one clinically possible). The wire is slowly withdrawn through the mouth until the end at the CTM disappears. At this point the wire-stiffener is advanced together with the tracheal tube. Once the tube is at an appropriate depth, both stiffener and wire are withdrawn and correct position of the tube confirmed by the tests outlined in Chapter 9. Withdrawal of the wire is always in this direction so that clean wire is drawn through the neck tissues, rather than wire coated with mouth commensals. Neck infections have resulted from the latter.

Fibreoptic-assisted technique

If the Cook retrograde kit is used, the cannula and J-wire are supplied and the wire will pass through the working channel of most intubating fibrescopes (but not the old Olympus LF-1). If the Cook kit is unavailable it is easy to substitute a standard 20-G cannula and find an appropriate size wire from the radiology suite. It needs to be at least 110 cm long, reasonably stiff and to be able to pass through the cannula and working channel of the fibrescope. A J-wire is not essential but can be helpful. An assistant is required during the procedure and prior mannikin practice is invaluable. The fibrescope,

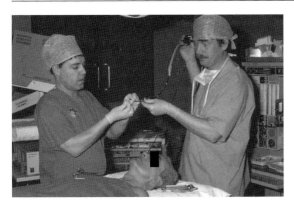

Figure 13.3 Retrograde – feeding wire into fibrescope channel.

preferably attached to closed circuit television (CCTV), should be ready and the tracheal tube loaded onto it but the light is turned off.

The technique starts in the same manner described above with preparation of the skin, appropriate local or general anaesthesia, puncture of the CTM by cannula and feeding of the wire cephalad. The cannula is left *in situ*. The wire is picked up in the pharynx, withdrawn from the mouth and passed through the working channel at the tip of the fibrescope until it emerges at the control section (Figure 13.3). With the light switched on the fibrescope (with loaded tube!) is advanced along the wire until the larynx is seen. Classically the scope slides over the wire, but sometimes the frictional forces mean that the scope and wire are slid 'down' together. Great care must be taken not to kink the wire.

Advancement of the scope under vision leads to the larynx and the tip of the cannula, which can now be removed. The scope is slid further down the wire until its tip is extremely close to the inner surface of the CTM. The wire is now withdrawn into the scope taking care not to allow the tip of the fibrescope to move far from the CTM. When the wire is within the scope the fibrescope can be manipulated further into the trachea and the tube railroaded as normal.

Variations

A number of variations have been described, often in single case reports. Puncture of the cricotracheal membrane rather than the CTM has been advocated. It is possible to place the fibrescope within the tube and feed the wire through the Murphy eye. The tube is slid down the wire until the larynx is visualized. Alternatively the wire and fibrescope can be placed independently within the tracheal tube. The advantage of these two variants is that the fibrescope does not run over the wire. A recent report describes the use of the Mini-Trach II. An incision is made with the knife in the CTM and the blue introducer is fed cephalad. The tube is advanced over the introducer in a traditional blind manner.

Key points

- Retrograde intubation has a high success rate with few complications.
- Commercial kits are available and can be placed on a difficult intubation trolley.
- Mannikin practice is useful and helpful.
- It can be used in the awake or anaesthetized patient.
- The fibreoptic-assisted variant is preferable because it is a visual technique.

Further reading

Audenaert SM, Montgomery CL, Stone B. Retrograde-assisted fiberoptic tracheal intubation in children with difficult airways. *Anesth Analg* 1991; **73**: 660–664.

Casthely PA, Landesman S, Fynaman PN. Retrograde intubation in patients undergoing open heart surgery. *Can Anaesth Soc J* 1985; **32**: 661–664.

Lechman MJ, Donahoo JS, Macvaugh H. Endotracheal intubation using percutaneous retrograde guidewire insertion followed by antegrade fibreoptic bronchoscopy. *Crit Care Med* 1986; **14**: 589–590.

Slots P, Vegger PB, Bettger H, Reinstrup P. Retrograde intubation with a Mini-Trach II kit. *Acta Anaesth Scand* 2003; **47**: 274–277.

Waters DJ. Guided blind endotracheal intubation. *Anaesthesia* 1963; **18**: 158–162.

A. Pearce

Thoracic surgical operations require the anaesthetist to be able to cease ventilation and allow deflation of the operative lung, to protect the lower lung from contamination with blood, tumour or infective material and to continue ventilation of the non-operative, dependent lung. Without the ability to separate and independently ventilate the lungs, thoracic surgery is hazardous. The first planned pulmonary resection by Block on a young female relative in 1883 was a disaster. She died on the operating table and Block committed suicide. A major component of safe thoracic anaesthesia is the appropriate use of endobronchial tubes, double-lumen tubes (DLTs) and bronchial blockers. Indications for their use are not restricted to pulmonary surgery and there are other clinical indications for lung separation (Table 14.1).

Endobronchial tubes

The first attempts at selective lung ventilation were with endobronchial tubes. These long, single-lumen

---

Table 14.1 Indications for lung separation

- Open pulmonary or pleural surgery
- Thoracoscopic procedures
- Unilateral pulmonary haemorrhage
- Unilateral pulmonary infection
- Thoracic vascular or gastrointestinal (GI) surgery
- Thoracic spine surgery (anterior approach)
- Bronchopleural fistula
- Tracheobronchial airway disruption
- Unilateral pulmonary lavage
- Independent lung ventilation in intensive care unit (ICU)

---

tubes were placed in the bronchus of the dependent, non-operative lung. The classical technique, devised by Magill, was to load the tube onto a rigid intubating bronchoscope and place the tube under direct bronchoscopic view. It was possible to ventilate both lungs at the end of surgery by withdrawing the endobronchial tube into the trachea. The technique of one-lung ventilation by endobronchial placement of a single-lumen tube is still in practice in specialized circumstances, usually with blind or fibreoptic positioning into the appropriate bronchus. The next development was of a combined tracheal tube and bronchial blocker (Macintosh–Leatherdale). This tube consisted of a standard tracheal tube and a cuffed blocker limb which entered the bronchus of the operative lung. Both lungs could be ventilated when the blocker cuff was deflated, and subsequent inflation of the cuff would isolate the operative lung. A long narrow channel through the blocker limb allowed egress of air and suctioning of blood or pus from the operative bronchus.

DLTs

Design

The first DLT was designed in 1949 by Carlens (1908–1990) for differential broncho-spirometry, prior to thoracic surgery. Carlens made a tube with two lumens, one longer tube passed into the left main bronchus and the other ended in the lower trachea. A carinal hook engaged the carina to allow and maintain correct placement. In his first study, Carlens inserted the DLT into 60 patients in the awake state under topical anaesthesia. His surgical colleagues at the Sabbatsberg Hospital, Sweden were so impressed that it was used in thoracic surgery with the first publication of its use in 500 lung resections in 1952.

There have been several designs over the years (Table 14.2) and a number of them (including the original Carlens) are available in single-use or disposable, red-rubber or polyvinyl chloride (PVC) material. The Robertshaw design proved particularly popular. Modern DLTs (Figure 14.1) are available as either left or right-sided (indicating the endobronchial component) in different sizes. Robertshaw ones are available in small, medium and large sizes, and the single-use PVC tubes are sized in French gauge (external circumference in mm) with 35 and 37 Fr being suitable for women and 39 and 41 Fr for males. Right-sided tubes have an orifice or slit (Figure 14.2) in the endobronchial portion (often in the cuff) which allows ventilation of the right upper lobe which arises usually 2.5 cm from the carina. No such orifice is needed on the left-sided tubes, as the left upper lobe arises approximately 5 cm from the carina.

Pre-insertion checks

Pre-insertion checks are to select the appropriate *size* and *side* tube, check inflation/deflation of the bronchial and tracheal cuffs and prepare the special Y-connector that allows connection of a twin-lumen tube to the breathing system. Insertion requires a good technique of direct laryngoscopy (picking up the epiglottis as required) to get the best view of the larynx, with a left-sided tube being introduced with a 90° clockwise orientation to position the angulated tip anteriorly. Once the tube is through the larynx, the stylet is removed and the tube advanced such that the lumens are side-by-side in the lower trachea to allow the endobronchial portion to enter the correct bronchus. Insertion depths are 29 cm at the teeth in the average male and 27 cm in the average female. There is some correlation between depth of insertion and height. Clamping one limb of the connector will stop ventilation of the lung on that side and opening of the cap will allow the lung to

Table 14.2 Eponymous equipment for thoracic anaesthesia

Endobronchial blocker
Magill
Vernon Thompson

Combined bronchus blocker and tracheal tube
Macintosh–Leatherdale

Endobronchial tubes
Magill
Machray
Green–Gordon
Brompton (Pallister)
Vellacott

DLTs
Carlens
Bryce–Smith
Bryce–Smith–Salt
White
Robertshaw

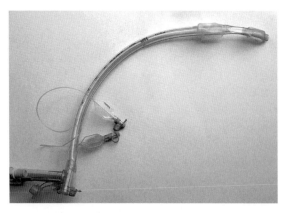

Figure 14.1 Portex right-sided DLT. *Note:* Blue bronchial limb, cuff and pilot balloon.

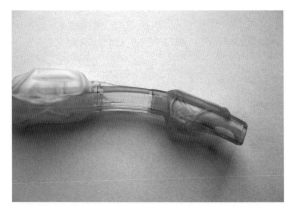

Figure 14.2 Opening in right bronchial limb cuff for upper lobe.

deflate when the pleura is open. The open cap allows a route for suctioning and placement of a flexible fibrescope for positioning purposes. It is generally easier to insert a left-sided DLT because of the difficulty presented by the position of the right upper lobe bronchus, but there are specific indications for a right-sided DLT (Table 14.3).

Checking position

Initially it should be confirmed that the DLT is in the respiratory, rather than the gastrointestinal (GI), tract by the methods described in Chapter 9. Then observations of chest movements are made when both lumens are patent and when, in turn, each limb of the Y-connector is clamped. Auscultation of the chest over the lobes should confirm the observation that clamping a limb leads to ipsilateral loss of ventilation with normal ventilation of all lobes of the contralateral lung. A suitable fibrescope should be available for checking or adjusting position of the DLT. Passing the fibrescope first through the tracheal limb allows the anaesthetist to confirm that

they have intubated the correct bronchus and that the depth of the tube is correct when a small amount of the blue bronchial cuff can be seen at the carina. With a right-sided DLT, the fibrescope should be placed also through the bronchial limb to make certain that the right upper lobe is aligned with the appropriate orifice in the tube.

There are a number of published reports of tracheo-bronchial tears due to DLTs, often due to initial overinflation or overdistension of the cuffs with nitrous oxide (N_2O). A review of the world literature published in 1999 identified 33 reports involving 46 patients. The authors made recommendations for safe placement of a DLT (Table 14.4).

Bronchial blockers

A bronchial blocker is effectively a small balloon on a long catheter with a central lumen which, when placed endobronchially, occludes ventilation on that side and allows egress of gas from the isolated lung. It is placed within the bronchus of the operative lung. Magill's version, in 1946, was placed under vision by rigid bronchoscopy, with a subsequent design by Thompson in 1947 becoming more popular, since it did not slip out of the bronchus so easily. Fogarty catheters may be used but current designs include the Univent tube (tracheal tube with a built-in adjustable blocker) and the Arndt blocker (Figure 14.3). DLTs are considerably more

---

Table 14.3 Indications for right-sided DLT

- Tumour in the left bronchus
- Left pneumonectomy
- Left lung transplantation
- Left tracheobronchial disruption
- Left bronchial stent *in situ*
- Distorted left bronchial anatomy

Table 14.4 Good practice recommendations for DLT placement

- Choose the largest PVC tube that will fit
- Remove the bronchial limb 'stylet' once the tip is passed the cords
- Advance the DLT to an appropriate distance (based on height)
- Check position clinically and with fibrescope
- Inflate cuffs slowly and carefully
- Keep intracuff pressures <30 cmH$_2$O
- Use a 3 ml syringe for bronchial cuff
- If N_2O used, fill cuffs with saline or N_2O/O_2 mix
- If N_2O used, check cuff pressures intermittently
- Deflate both cuffs before removing or repositioning the tube
- Deflate bronchial cuff when not needed

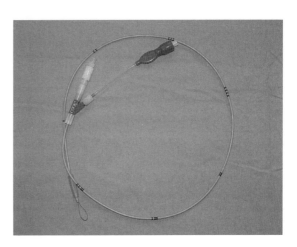

Figure 14.3 Arndt bronchial blocker.

Table 14.5 Relative indications for bronchial blocker over DLT

- Abnormal tracheo-bronchial anatomy
- Difficult intubation
- Tracheostomy tube *in situ*
- Paediatric patients
- When postoperative ventilation planned
- When patient ventilated preoperatively

Table 14.6 Steps in placement of Arndt bronchial blocker

- Check which size tracheal tube needed
- Intubate with appropriate single-lumen tube
- Attach multiport connector
- Ventilate patient through breathing port
- Place fibrescope through its port
- Place blocker through its port
- Thread fibrescope through blocker loop (Figure 14.4)
- Pass fibrescope into appropriate bronchus
- Slide blocker off fibrescope into position
- Withdraw fibrescope into trachea and check blocker position
- Remove blocker loop only when correctly placed

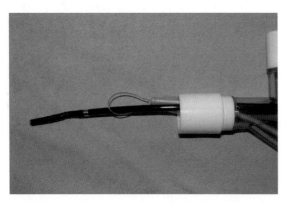

Figure 14.4 Passing fibrescope through loop.

popular and convenient than bronchial blockers in thoracic anaesthesia, but there are a number of indications (Table 14.5) where a bronchial blocker is preferable and there is a resurgence of interest in them. This is partly due to the design of the Arndt blocker which allows easy placement under vision with a fibrescope and has a connector which allows continued ventilation through the tracheal tube while placement is in progress, and due to the simplicity of the Univent tube which is available in all sizes from baby to adult. The steps in placement of an Arndt blocker are given in Table 14.6 and information on the Internet is available for both the Univent and Arndt systems.

Key points

- Lung isolation is useful in pulmonary and non-pulmonary surgery.
- DLTs are usually simple, quick and effective.
- DLT placement should be confirmed clinically and endoscopically.
- Bronchial blockers (an old technique) are increasingly popular.
- Bronchial blockers have several advantages over DLTs.

Further reading

Arndt blocker on www.cookgroup.com/cook_critical_care/blocker.html

Fitzmaurice BG, Brodsky JB. Airway rupture from double-lumen tubes. *J Cardiothor Vasc Anesth* 1999; **13**: 322–329.

Klein U *et al*. Role of fiberoptic bronchoscopy in conjunction with the use of double-lumen tubes for thoracic anaesthesia. *Anesthesiology* 1998; **88**: 346–350.

Univent tube on www.vitaid.com/usa/univent/index.htm

'DIFFICULT AIRWAYS': CAUSATION AND PREDICTION

15

I. Calder

Defining, describing and identifying 'difficult' airways are difficult tasks. The obviously problematic patients are, in a sense, no problem, since everybody understands the situation and suitable tactics, staff and equipment can be deployed. The majority of difficult patients that anaesthetists encounter look 'more-or-less' normal. We are still unable to identify these patients with acceptable accuracy. Anaesthetists must be prepared to adapt their technique if difficulty occurs.

There can be no doubt that the advent of the laryngeal mask airway (LMA) has decreased the frequency of difficulty with the airway. Many patients who would have been intubated have an LMA instead, so that episodes of difficult laryngoscopy are avoided, and when difficult laryngoscopy is encountered an LMA is often used instead of a tracheal tube.

Having found a difficult airway, it is by no means easy to describe the problem in a way which will be of practical help to subsequent anaesthetists. It has been shown that most anaesthetists ignore a history of difficult intubation, which may be because the problem was not accurately defined or they believe that they can do better. Many scoring systems have been proposed, but the only one that has stood the test of time is Cormack and Lehane's description of direct laryngoscopy.

Causes of difficulty

Non-patient factors

Whether you will experience difficulty with an airway will depend on:

a Who you are

b Where you are
c What equipment and drugs you have
d Who you have to help you
e What the patient is like

One can perm the factors above to demonstrate that difficulty with an airway can occur with any patient. Any practitioner undertaking to anaesthetize a patient must consider whether he/she has the appropriate expertise, drugs, equipment, assistance, and whether the environment is suitable (inducing anaesthesia in a non-hospital setting, or even in an unfamiliar part of a hospital can be very stressful). Beyond a minimum standard, the equipment and drugs required are a matter of debate. Should a fibreoptic laryngoscope and/or equipment for transtracheal jet ventilation (TTJV) be available in all locations? Opinions vary. A separate system for inflating the patient's lungs (such as an airway mask breathing unit, AMBU, bag) should always be available.

Which drugs should be regarded as essential will also provoke debate. For instance, many practitioners feel that succinylcholine should be drawn up before the administration of any anaesthetic. Others regard this as wasteful.

Patient factors

How you approach a classification of the causes of difficulty with the airway depends on whether you are trying to answer a question in an examination, or formulate a strategy to deal with a particular patient. In the examination setting an aetiological approach is helpful, while in day-to-day practice a procedural analysis is appropriate.

Airway difficulty	
Aetiological	**Procedural**
Reflexes	Mask
Stiffness	LMA
Deformity	Laryngoscopy
Swelling	Intubation
Foreign bodies	Tracheotomy
'High tariff'	

Causes of airway difficulty

Aetiological classification

In attempting to remember and classify all the causes of difficulty one can apply the usual patho-logical sieves such as 'congenital/acquired' and 'in the lumen, in the wall and outside the wall'. No system is perfect.

Reflexes

Unwanted reflexes provide the common airway problems. The 'submarine analogy' (that in general safety can be found at moderate depths) is a useful guide to safe anaesthesia. Laryngospasm, coughing, breath holding, and regurgitation occur at light levels of anaesthesia. Failure to adequately suppress airway reflexes before instrumentation is dangerous.

Stiffness/deformity

Anaesthesia becomes hazardous when the standard airway clearing manoeuvres of jaw thrust and head tilt cannot be applied because of immobility of the tissues. Deformity is often allied to stiffness. The arthritides are obvious examples. Other examples are Klippel–Feil, Pierre–Robin and Treacher–Collins deformities, ankylosing spondylitis, sclero-derma, burn or radiotherapy contractures and cranio-cervical fixation devices. Muscular rigidity in status, tetanus or rabies could be included here. Unusual causes include oral sub-mucous fibrosis in betel nut chewers and joint stiffness in diabetes mellitus.

Swelling

The commonest problem is obesity, although even gross obesity is not a good predictor of airway

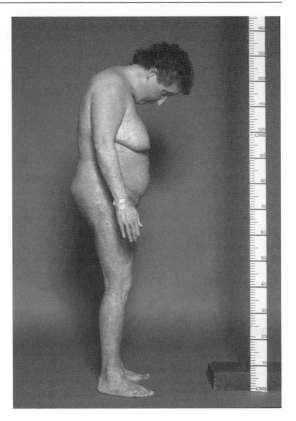

Figure 15.1 Stiffness and deformity (Psoriaritic arthropathy causing cervical flexion deformity). Courtesy of Mr A. Crockard.

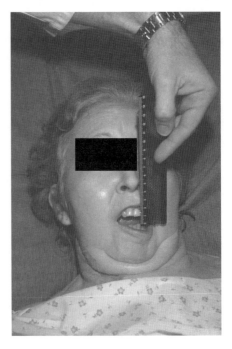

Figure 15.2 Stiffness. Rheumatoid arthritis affecting cervical spine and temporomandibular joints.

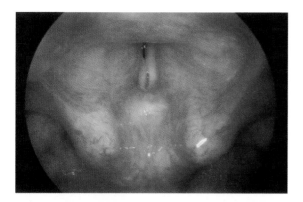

Figure 15.3 Swelling and stiffness. Glottic rheumatoid arthritis. The arytenoids and ary-epiglottic folds are swollen, and the airway is narrow. (Reprinted, with permission from Benjamin B. *Endolaryngeal Surgery*. Martin Dunitz, London 1998.)

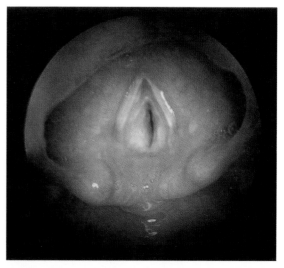

Figure 15.5 Swelling. Laryngo-tracheo-bronchitis. (Reprinted, with permission from Benjamin B. *Endolaryngeal Surgery*. Martin Dunitz, London 1998.)

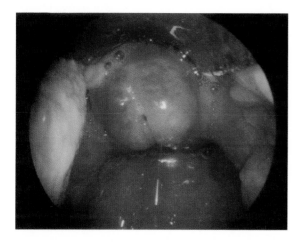

Figure 15.4 Swelling. Epiglottitis in a child. (Reprinted, with permission from Benjamin B. *Endolaryngeal Surgery*. Martin Dunitz, London 1998.)

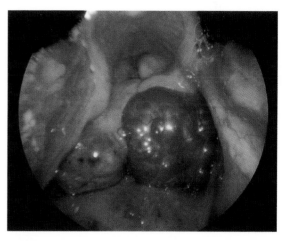

Figure 15.6 Swelling. Cavernoma causing airway obstruction. (Reprinted, with permission from Benjamin B. *Endolaryngeal Surgery*. Martin Dunitz, London 1998.)

difficulty. Other causes include infections, such as epiglottitis or Ludwig's angina, tumours, trauma (including post-surgical oedema or haematoma); airway obstruction from neck swelling due to leaking irrigation fluid during prolonged shoulder joint arthroscopy, and cerebrospinal fluid after cervical spine surgery have both been described, acromegaly, inflammation such as rheumatoid arthritis, and anaphylaxis. Lingual tonsils can cause unexpected difficulty. Thyroid and mediastinal tumours can present problems both at induction and recovery from anaesthesia, since

the excision of a tumour can leave a weakened trachea unsupported.

Foreign bodies

Accidental inhalation of objects placed in the mouth is not confined to children. Alcohol is often, but by no means always a factor in adults. Aspiration of solids and liquids at induction of anaesthesia is dealt with in Chapter 20. Practitioners vary in their policy

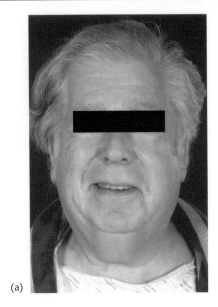 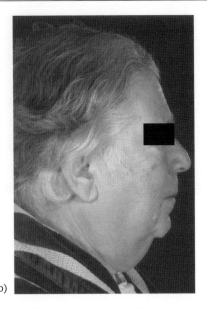

(a)   (b)

Figure 15.7 Unidentified difficult airway. This patient presented for a ureteroscopy. No relevant airway history. Mallampati II, IDD 3.7 cm, B protrusion, thyro-mental distance 10 cm. It was difficult to maintain an airway with either face mask and airway or a size 4 or 5 LMA. Direct laryngoscopy was Grade 3.

about full or partial dentures. Removing dentures can make mask anaesthesia and laryngoscopy difficult (a gap in the incisors has this effect) and isolated teeth may damage gums or be displaced themselves. The author's policy is to leave dentures in, unless the patient prefers to have them out (which many do). It is worth noting that most dentures are radiolucent.

'High tariff' patients

The purpose of this division is to try and include those patients in whom some factor is present that makes the management of the airway more of a problem for the anaesthetist. The reader can formulate their own list. The author would include: uncooperative patients, full stomach – particularly obstetric patients, no venous access, very important persons (VIPs) and other 'precious' patients. The effect is to limit the options open to the anaesthetist and to increase his/her stress level. That excessive stress can degrade performance was first proposed in 1908 by Yerkes and Dodson, who observed an inverted U-shaped curve when performance in a maze was plotted against increasing stress (electric shocks) in rats. There is evidence to suggest that

the effect is accentuated as the complexity of the task increases.

Two classic difficult airways:

Rheumatoid arthritis	Acromegaly
Cranio-cervical junction involved	Tissue hypertrophy
	Glottis involved: stenosis can occur
Temporo-mandibular joint involved	
Glottis involved: stenosis can occur	
Direct laryngoscopy often difficult	Mask anaesthesia can be difficult
Fibreoptic intubation can be difficult if the glottis is displaced from midline	Direct laryngoscopy can be difficult
	Fibreoptic laryngoscopy can be difficult
Stridor common on extubation – use a small tube	Complete obstruction on extubation has been recorded – use a small tube

Procedural classification

Mask anaesthesia

Professor Benumof's suggested definition of having to use two hands to control the airway, with an assistant squeezing the bag, and oral and nasal airways *in situ*, seems a practical one. Such difficulty is, fortunately, rare. Minor (though troublesome) degrees of difficulty are encountered with bearded or edentulous patients. Patients with large faces (e.g. acromegaly) can be a problem. Gross obesity is a weak predictor.

Difficult LMA insertion

A satisfactory airway can be established with an LMA in approximately 99.8% of patients. Insertion becomes more difficult, when mouth opening is restricted. The lower limit of normal mouth opening in young adults is 3.7 cm, but an LMA can be inserted with about 2.5 cm of inter-incisor distance. If there is doubt the procedure should be performed awake, using topical anaesthesia.

Difficult direct laryngoscopy

We often call this phenomenon 'difficult intubation', but strictly speaking we are incorrect; a *difficult* direct laryngoscopy patient may be *easily* intubated with a fibreoptic endoscope. The term 'anterior larynx' used to be applied when a line of sight could not be established, but it has been supplanted by grading systems. The most widely used system was proposed by Cormack and Lehane in 1984 (Figure 15.8). Grades 3 (only epiglottis visible) and 4 (no glottic structure visible) are regarded as 'difficult'. The prevalence of difficulty varies from about 2% in a general surgical population to almost 50% in patients with rheumatoid cervical spine disease. The Cormack and Lehane system is attractive from the practical point of view, since it correlates with the envelope of use of the gum-elastic (Eschmann) bougie. Nearly all Grade 2 (arytenoids cartilages visible) and many Grade 3 glottises can be intubated with the aid of a gum-elastic bougie. A weakness of the Cormack grading is the breadth of significance of a Grade 2 view. Some Grade 2 glottises are by no means easy to intubate, a gum-elastic bougie is often required. The division of Grade 2 into 2a (part of cords visible and 2b (only arytenoids visible)) is a sensible modification. An alternative descriptive system, the

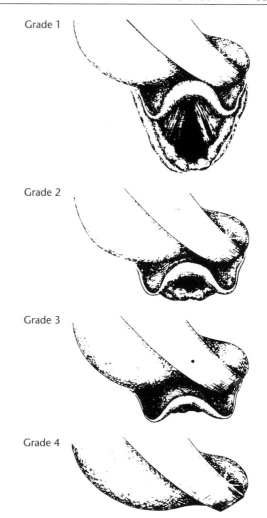

Figure 15.8 Cormack and Lehane Score. (Reprinted, with permission from Williams KN, Carli F, Cormack RS. *Br J Anaesth* 1991; **66**: 38–44.)

POGO (Percentage Of Glottic Opening) score was proposed by Ochroch and colleagues, but it is not in common use.

Difficult fibreoptic laryngoscopy

Blood, or other fluids in the airway are the chief causes of difficulty. Lateral displacement of the glottis, as is sometimes seen in rheumatoid arthritis can be a problem, and tissue swelling that occludes the air space will prevent vision. Difficulty has been reported in anaesthetized acromegalic patients for this reason.

Difficult intubation

As mentioned above this term tends to be used synonymously with difficult direct laryngoscopy. 'True' difficult intubation despite a good view of the glottis is rare, although difficulty is often artificially induced in the author's experience when an unnecessarily large tube is used, which obtunds the view of the glottic opening as it is advanced. It is rarely necessary to use a tube of larger than 7.0 mm inner diameter for anaesthesia. Larger sizes may be advantageous in intensive care. True difficult intubation occurs when the glottis or trachea is stenosed in disease processes such as tumours, epiglottitis, rheumatoid arthritis and acromegaly. Difficult intubation has been defined in terms of number of attempts or elapsed time. Benumof has pointed out that these parameters may not be applicable in the case of a sensible decision to make only one or even no attempt when difficulty is obvious. Benumof proposed that a definition could be *failure despite an optimal best attempt.*

Difficult tracheostomy/ostomy

Flexion deformity or severe shortening of the cervical spine can render tracheostomy impossible. Anterior cervical swelling or large cervical tumours can also make surgical access difficult or impossible.

Common meanings of 'difficult airways'

Difficult intubation

- Inability to intubate within a certain time (American Society of Anesthesiologists (ASA), 10 min).
- Inability to intubate within a number of attempts at direct laryngoscopy (ASA, 3).
- Cormack and Lehane Grade 3 or 4 view of larynx (epiglottis only or no laryngeal structures).
- Requirement for additional equipment (other than traditional laryngoscope).

Difficult ventilation

- Inability to keep oxygen saturations >90% with 100% oxygen by facemask or reverse signs of inadequate ventilation (ASA).
- Catastrophic failure of mask ventilation leads to morbidity or mortality. 'Problematic' facemask ventilation in which more than one person may be needed or problems might arise if facemask ventilation is required for some time.

Pre-anaesthetic identification of airway difficulty

Enthusiasm about this subject has undergone a swing from initial optimism to near despair. Unfortunately, it seems that we can only reliably identify the difficult patients who have gross abnormalities. We can also expect to be able to identify most of the difficult patients, who suffer from a disease known to be associated with difficulty. At the time of writing it must be admitted that we cannot reliably identify the difficult cases in the general population who look more-or-less normal and have no history, such as the case illustrated in Figure 15.6.

Difficult direct laryngoscopy

Prediction of airway difficulty is generally taken to mean difficulty with direct laryngoscopy, because that is the common difficulty encountered in day-to-day practice. A number of predictive tests have been described (such as Mallampati, thyro-mental, sterno-mental, ABC protrusion – A: lower incisors anterior to upper; B: edge to edge; C: lower incisors unable to touch uppers, Wilson risk sum), all of which have yielded disappointing results when applied as screening tests to healthy populations (Table 15.1).

Difficult mask ventilation

Ideally, we would like to identify patients who will be difficult to mask ventilate, since that is much more dangerous than difficult direct laryngoscopy. However, since true difficulty in an apparently normal patient is so rare, it is not possible to do so. Minor difficulty is common, but predictive testing systems have proved disappointing even for this.

Sensitivity, specificity and positive predictive value

Discussion of this subject is bedeviled by the difficulty encountered by most of us in understanding the terminology used to describe the results of studies. Nearly everybody finds the concepts of sensitivity, specificity and positive predictive value (PPV) confusing at times. The reader may care to read the excellent article by Loong in the *British*

Table 15.1 Results of Mallampati examination trials

Study	Patients	N	Difficult Direct laryngoscopy (%)	Sensitivity	Specificity	PPV	LR
Cohen	General	667	7	62	95	28	13
Frerk	General	244	4.5	81	82	17	4.5
Oates	General	675	1.8	42	84	4	2.6
Rocke	Obstetrics	1500	1.6	59	74	4	2.2
Butler	General	220	8.2	56	81	21	2.9
Savva	General	350	4.9	65	66	9	1.4
Tse	General	471	13	66	65	22	1.8
Ganzouri	General	10507	6.1	45	89	21	4
Schmitt	Acromegaly	128	25	44	76	32	1.8
Calder	Cervical	253	20	56	96	78	14

The results for the other tests are rather worse; those for the sterno-mental distance were described by Farmery as indicating that the test had *'an accuracy approaching worthlessness.'*

Medical Journal (BMJ), which gave not only an excellent explanation of the terms, but also an example of the difficulties, as he himself mixed up the terms, which led to extensive correspondence.

What we want in a predictive test is that it should be sensitive (sensitivity: positivity in disease) and have a high positive predictive value (PPV: the proportion of positive results that turn out to be correct). A high PPV depends largely on the test having a high specificity (specificity: negativity in health). Unfortunately it is the case that high sensitivity and high specificity do not go together, so that either we tend to have a test that declares an aggravating number of false predictions or one that misses many true positives.

Effect of prevalence on PPV of a test with a sensitivity of 50%, and specificity of 70% (e.g. the Mallampati – see Table 15.1)

(a) *Prevalence = 2%*

Number of positive test results = 1 true positive + 29.4 false positives (30% of 98 healthy subjects = 29.4).

PPV = 1/30.4 = **3.2%**

(b) *Prevalence = 50%*

Number of positive test results = 25 true positives + 15 false positives.

PPV = 25/40 = **62.5%**

Prevalence is important

We need to keep the likely prevalence of the problem in the population being studied in mind, because any test will, for a given sensitivity and specificity, have a much better PPV when the prevalence is high.

The conditions we are concerned with such as difficult direct laryngoscopy have a low prevalence (about 2%) in an unselected surgical population. The dangerous condition of difficult mask ventilation is rare (about 1:7 of difficult direct laryngoscopies), so that predictive methods are inaccurate.

Likelihood ratios

It is very hard to juggle with values of sensitivity and specificity in one's head and apply them to an individual patient. The difficulty of working with sensitivity and specificity can be decreased by using the likelihood ratio (LR = sensitivity/1 − specificity). The LR can be used to calculate the increase in probability of a correct diagnosis provided by a positive test result. The pre-test probability is the prevalence of the problem in the population being studied. The post-test probability is numerically the same as the PPV. Nomograms are available in evidence based medicine texts (Figure 15.9). The effect of prevalence can be appreciated by plotting different lines. If we could devise a test of 100%

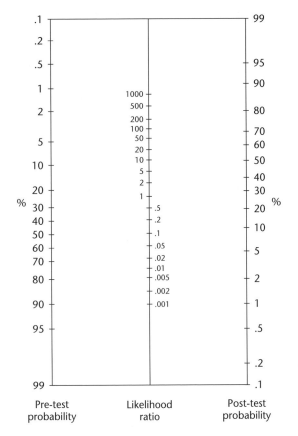

Figure 15.9 Nomogram for plotting increase in probability. (Reprinted with permission from Sacket DL *et al. Clinical Epidemiology: A Basic Science for Clinical Medicine*, 2nd edition. Boston/Toronto: Little Brown and Company, 1991.)

sensitivity and 99.5% specificity (LR = 200) we can still only expect about 75% of predictions to be correct when the prevalence is 2%, but more than 95% of predictions will be correct if the prevalence is 20% (Figure 15.9).

What pre-anaesthetic airway assessment should be performed?

Yentis wrote an important editorial in *Anaesthesia*, questioning the 'pointless ritual' of airway examination. However, he did not suggest that we abandon our attempts. It is in the nature of things that should an airway problem occur, it will tend to reflect badly on the practitioner if an assessment has not been done, however inaccurate our methods have been shown to be.

It is interesting to compare the evolution of thinking about airway examination with that about other screening programmes. The attempts to screen for breast, cervical and prostate cancer are similarly controversial. The idea that screening symptomless patients is a good thing, so that treatment can be started early, seems obvious. However, the problems of false negatives and positives are serious, and evidence that mortality is reduced is disputed. The view that screening programmes should not be adopted until benefit is proved seems to be gaining ground (see screening without evidence of efficacy. bmj.com 2004. http://bmj.bmjjournals.com/cgi/content/full/328/7435/301).

It is indisputably necessary to obtain any history available from the patient or records, and to examine the patients' dentition and establish that the inter-dental distance is normal. Beyond that, it can be argued that it is pointless to do anything else, unless the patient has a risk factor, such as a disease associated with difficulty. When the patient has risk factors it is reasonable to try and increase the probability of a diagnosis of easiness or difficulty. The concept of the Mallampati examination remains attractive, in that how far one can see down the airway without a laryngoscope should have some bearing on what will be seen at laryngoscopy. The examination is very subjective and the grades are imprecisely described in the literature. There is probably only a need for a 'bad' and a 'not bad' grade, which each practitioner evolves for him/herself. There is no justification for continuing to use Samsoon and Young's four-grade modification.

History

Any information gained from the patient, relatives or hospital records is very valuable. Conditions can improve, but in general get worse, as the mobility of the cervical spine and temporo-mandibular joints decrease with age, so a record of easiness is no guarantee.

A history of any of the conditions known to be associated with difficulty places the patient in a different risk group. Specific questions may be necessary, such as about intermittent hoarseness and stridor in rheumatoid arthritis and acromegaly (glottic involvement) or obstructive sleep apneoa in acromegaly and obesity.

Examination

Any feature that may make mask anaesthesia difficult is of particular interest. Beards in themselves are a nuisance and may camouflage jaw abnormalities, while edentulous faces are hard to seal masks to.

The particular points of interest are given below:

Airway patency

Stridor indicates severe airway obstruction. Patients with supra-glottic obstruction may not have stridor despite severe obstruction (e.g. cervical haematoma/oedema). Severe tracheal obstruction has been mistaken for asthma.

Mouth opening

A minimum of normality of 3.7 cm has been suggested in young adults. However, we do not know at what measurement airway difficulty can be expected. At 2.5 cm it will be difficult to insert an LMA. Measuring inter-dental distance will, in practice, be mostly done by eye, with formal measurement undertaken when abnormality is suspected. The ability to protrude the mandible is also of interest, since jaw thrust and direct laryngoscopy both require protrusion. An ABC classification, or protrusion can be assessed in termsof the ability of the patient to bite his/her upper lip. Grade C protrusion is rare but diagnostic for difficult laryngoscopy. Unfortunately, Grade B has poor PPV.

Cranio-cervical mobility

Head tilt and direct laryngoscopy both require extension at the cranio-cervical junction – the occipito-atlanto-axial complex. Some flexion of the spine below C3 (the sniffing position – occiput raised about 10 cm) is helpful in difficult cases (sometimes even greater flexion can be helpful). Clinical assessment is difficult, as in practice it is hard to distinguish cranio–cervical movement from total cervical

movement, and because the normal range of cranio-cervical and total cervical flexion/extension changes with age and what represents significant abnormality is uncertain. Wilson suggested placing a pencil on the patient's forehead and observing the angle swept by the pencil between flexion and extension. Less than 80° being considered abnormal. Curiously, the Mallampati emerged as the best predictor of difficulty in a study of patients with cervical spine disease. It has been shown recently in conscious volunteers that mouth opening is related to cranio-cervical flexion/extension. About 26° of extension is required to allow full mouth opening and if extension beyond the neutral position is prevented 95% of subjects have an inter-dental distance of less than 3.7 cm. Restricted mouth opening may be due to cranio-cervical rigidity, which provides a basis for the success of the Mallampati in patients with restricted cranio-cervical mobility.

Dr Mallampati's examination

- Described in 1985 – three grades.
- Fourth grade added by Samsoon and Young – not evidence based.
- Only two grades are required.
- Serious inter-observer variability.
- PPV has only exceeded 50% in one study.
- Remains a logical approach.
- Not suitable as a screening test.

Thyro- and sterno-mental distance

- Similar to Mallampati in being unsuitable for screening.
- Accuracy can be improved by correcting for height and weight.

Combining tests

- First suggested by Frerk.
- Not successful in a low prevalence population.
- Sensible practice in a high prevalence population.

Investigations

Investigations are rarely indicated, but computerized tomography (CT) scans of the mediastinum can give useful information about the extent of tracheal deformation. In patients with cervical spine disease cervical radiographs or scans can give an indication of the likelihood of difficulty. If the disease process involves the upper three vertebrae, difficulty is likely. Preliminary flexible fibreoptic laryngoscopy is sensible when a glottic or sub-glottic lesion is suspected.

> **Recommended routine assessment**
>
> - A history of disease associated with difficulty, or of actual anaesthetic difficulty should always be sought.
> - Adequacy of mouth opening should be sought in all patients. Less than 37 mm falls outside the normal range
> - Attempt to assess cranio-cervical movement. This remains a difficult task. In the author's opinion some indication of restriction can be gained by observing head movement during maximum mouth opening.

Key points

- Serious airway difficulty is rare in healthy patients.
- 'Screening' a healthy population is unrewarding.
- All methods of prediction perform more successfully when the prevalence of difficulty is high – in diseases known to be associated with difficulty.
- In all patients – history, inter-dental distance, dentition.
- The Mallampati examination is unsuitable as a screening test, has poor inter-observer concordance and more than two grades are unnecessary. Maximum mouth opening can be used to identify poor cranio-cervical extension.
- Unexpected difficulty with an airway is a fact of anaesthetic life.

Further reading

Benumof JL. Definition and incidence of the difficult airway. In: Benumof JL, (Ed.) *Airway Management – Principles and Practice*. St Louis: Mosby, 1996: 121–125.

Calder I, Picard J, Chapman M, O'Sullevan C, Crockard HA. Mouth opening – a new angle. *Anesthesiology* 2003; **99**: 799–801.

Crosby ET, Cooper RM, Douglas MJ *et al.* The unanticipated difficult airway with recommendations for management. *Can J Anaesth* 1998; **45**: 757–776.

Karkouti K, Rose DK, Ferris LE, Wigglesworth DF, Meisani-Fard T, Lee H. Inter-observer reliability of ten tests used for predicting difficult tracheal intubation. *Can J Anaesth* 1996; **43**: 541–543.

Landtwing K. Evaluation of the normal range of mandibular opening in children and adolescents with special reference to age and stature. *J Maxillofac Surg* 1978; **6**: 157–162.

Langeron O, Masso E, Huraux C *et al.* Prediction of difficult mask ventilation. *Anesthesiology* 2000; **92**: 1229–1236.

Law M. Screening without evidence of efficacy. *Br Med J* 2004; **328**: 301–302.

Loong T-W. Understanding sensitivity and specificity with the right side of the brain. *Br Med J* 2003; **327**: 716–719.

McGovern DPB, Valori RM, Summerskill WSM, Levi M. Evidence based medicine. Oxford: Bios Scientific Publishers Ltd, 2001.

Ovassapian A, Glassenberg R, Randel GI *et al.* The unexpected difficult airway and lingual tonsil hyperplasia. *Anesthesiology* 2002; **97**: 124–132.

Rose DK, Cohen MM. The airway: problems and predictions in 18,500 patients. *Can J Anaesth* 1994; **41**: 372–383.

Sjoberg H. Interaction of task difficulty, activation, and workload. *J Human Stress* 1977; **3**: 33–38.

Tham EJ, Gildersleve CD, Sanders LD, Mapleson WW, Vaughan RS. Effects of posture, phonation, and observer on Mallampati classification. *Br J Anaesth* 1992; **68**: 32–38.

Yarrow S, Hare J, Robinson KN. Recent trends in tracheal intubation: a retrospective analysis. *Anaesthesia* 2003; **58**: 1019–1022.

Yentis SM. Predicting difficult intubation – worthwhile exercise or pointless ritual? *Anaesthesia* 2002; **57**: 105–109.

Yentis SM, Lee DJ. Evaluation of an improved scoring system for the grading of direct laryngoscopy. *Anaesthesia* 1998; **53**: 1041–1044.

THE PAEDIATRIC AIRWAY 16

R.W.M. Walker

Anatomical and physiological differences

At birth the human larynx is well developed for the demands of life and the neonate is capable of breathing, limited phonation, and airway protection during feeding. The larynx lies opposite the third cervical vertebra and the epiglottis is long and curled, often in the classical Ω shape and is in frequent contact with the soft palate during the first 6 months of age. This allows for feeding and breathing to occur simultaneously by interlocking of these structures, creating lateral channels for feeding and a central passage for breathing via the nasal airway. This situation lasts for 12–18 months. The tongue is large relative to the mandibular space and fills the oral cavity, allowing the tongue to protrude during feeding. Infants are preferential nasal breathers and the presence of nasal obstruction (e.g. choanal atresia) can cause significant airway problems.

The subglottic area in the term-baby is funnel shaped from the top down and the posterior lamina of the cricoid ring is tilted back and inferiorly making it particularly susceptible to trauma during endotracheal intubation. The smaller size of the paediatric airway means that a small decrease in diameter may cause significant airway obstruction. The cricoid ring is the narrowest part of the child's airway. The length of the trachea in the newborn is 5–6 cm and increases during the first year of life to about 8 cm. The epiglottis moves away from the soft palate at around 6 months and the tongue descends into the pharynx at about 1 year of age allowing greater phonation. The differences between

the infant and the older child's skull can be seen in Figure 16.1. The infant has a larger occiput and the base of skull has a much lesser concavity. This pattern persists for the first year of life but by the age of 6 years has developed the deep concave configuration (see Figure 16.1) of the adult base of skull. These changes have relevance when choosing laryngoscope blades and with positioning of the head and neck during laryngoscopy. The large occiput negates the need for a pillow to place the patient into the 'sniffing the morning air' position.

Neonates and babies cope poorly with airway obstruction because of a high oxygen consumption and inefficient mechanics of respiration. Oxygen consumption in the neonate is approximately $7\,ml\,kg^{-1}\,min^{-1}$ and this decreases gradually during childhood to the adult value of $3.5\,ml\,kg^{-1}\,min^{-1}$. The higher oxygen requirement means that airway obstruction or apnoea will produce hypoxia more rapidly in children than adults. Infants have a fixed tidal volume and are diaphragmatic breathers, responding to airway obstruction by increasing respiratory rate. They have fewer type I fatigue-resistant fibres and are therefore prone to fatigue. Infants are therefore susceptible to airway obstruction, hypoxia and the effects of hypoxia.

Relevance of these differences

During the use of a face mask in neonates and infants, airway obstruction can be caused by injudicious placement of the fingers on the base of the tongue causing the tongue to be forced against the palate obstructing the airway. This is made worse by the edentulous nature of the infant. A face mask

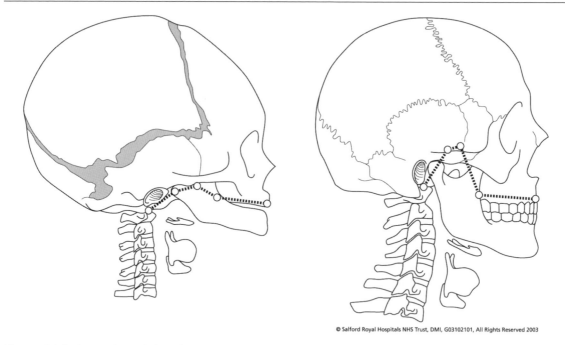

Figure 16.1 Comparison of the infant and older child skulls, showing the differences in shape, concavity of skull base and position of airway structures.

must be placed carefully on to the face and the mouth kept slightly open. Endotracheal intubation can be hampered by anatomical differences already mentioned. The epiglottis in infants is large, floppy and Ω shaped. It makes an angle of 45° with the base of the tongue and overhangs the glottis. The proximity of the larynx and the tongue causes an acute angle between the lingual and glottic axes making visualization of the glottis and intubation difficult.

Selection of laryngoscope blade

The use of a curved blade is less useful in the infant because there exists relative macroglossia, so that the displacement/compression of the tongue into the mandibular space to reveal the larynx is more difficult and is exacerbated by any degree of micrognathia. Straight-bladed laryngoscopes take up less space in the mouth and can be used to lift the epiglottis and provide clear views of the glottis, particularly when used by a 'paraglossal' approach (Figure 16.2). The infant McCoy laryngoscope blade is another option.

Cuffed or uncuffed endotracheal tubes in paediatric practice

Traditionally, uncuffed tracheal tubes are used up to the age of 9–10 years. The rationale for this is that an uncuffed tube of appropriate size will fit 'snugly' at the level of the cricoid ring, protecting the airway and allowing ventilation with only a minimal leak. The leak is used to judge that the tube is not too large. Laryngeal damage from the placement of uncuffed tubes is associated generally with the placement of too large a tube and occurs at the level of the cricoid region in the postero-lateral region. A cuff is unnecessary in routine general anaesthesia and can cause significant damage either due to damage of the tracheal mucosa lower in the mid-trachea or due to incorrect placement of the cuff, either in the cricoid region or at the level of the larynx itself. Recently, cuffed tubes have appeared in paediatric practice but they remain controversial and are limited to specific clinical areas. In the paediatric intensive care unit (PICU), a child with poor lung compliance can be difficult or impossible to ventilate adequately due to a

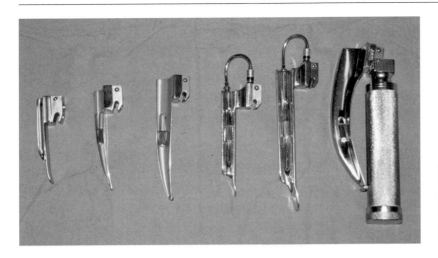

Figure 16.2 A selection of laryngoscope blades used in paediatric practice. From the left they are the infant Miller, Robert–Shaw, Magill and lastly the MacIntosh.

variable leak around an uncuffed tube. Leaks can also cause difficulties in accurate respiratory monitoring and may be implicated in silent pulmonary aspiration.

Paediatric airway problems

Paediatric practice can produce some of the most difficult airway problems that an anaesthetist can experience. There are well-known syndromes, such as Pierre–Robin, Treacher–Collins or Hunter–Hurler, that will challenge even the most experienced practitioner. The fact that 'awake' intubation or regional procedures are rarely alternatives in paediatric practice adds to the difficulty. The rapidity of oxygen desaturation in children is frightening. However, unlike adults, a normal-looking child will very rarely prove to be a difficult laryngoscopy. If difficulty is anticipated there should be, in general, two anaesthetists present at induction. A particularly serious situation may develop during an inhalational induction before intravenous access is established. If the airway is lost due to laryngeal spasm, suxamethonium may be administered intramuscularly, intralingually or via the intraosseous route.

Airway obstruction

There are a number of causes of airway obstruction in the child (Table 16.1). Infants <5 months old are preferential nasal breathers and obstruction of both nasal passages can cause significant obstruction.

The chest wall, trachea and bronchi in an infant are pliable so the calibre of the extrathoracic airways depends on the balance between intraluminal pressure and atmospheric pressure. Inspiratory efforts to overcome an extrathoracic obstruction generate large negative intrapleural pressures and these are transmitted to the extrathoracic airway as significant negative intraluminal pressures. The result is that atmospheric pressure around the extrathoracic airway causes dynamic compression (collapse) of the airway during inspiration, resulting in inspiratory stridor (noisy breathing). The application of continuous positive airway pressure (CPAP) helps splint the airway open. The patency of lower intrathoracic airways depends on the balance of intraluminal and intrapleural pressures. Large positive intrapleural pressures generated during active expiration cause dynamic compression of the airways downstream of the obstruction, so that intrathoracic obstructions cause expiratory stridor. Agitation and crying make dynamic airway compression worse. The diaphragm and intercostal muscles in infants have fewer fatigue resistant type I fibres. If the work of breathing increases respiratory failure sets in quickly.

Intubation of the child with airway obstruction

A provisional diagnosis should be made by the paediatric team and the at-risk child treated and monitored in a high dependency unit. Early involvement of the ENT (ear, nose and throat) and anaesthetic

Table 16.1 Causes of airway obstruction in the child

Congenital	Acquired
Choanal atresia	Epiglottitis
Laryngomalacia	Laryngotracheobronchitis
Subglottic stenosis	Bacterial tracheitis
Subglottic haemangioma	Subglottic stenosis
Webs	Burns
Cysts	Peritonsillar abscess
Tracheal stenosis	Foreign body
Vascular rings or slings	Angioneurotic oedema
Bilateral vocal cord paralysis	Nerve palsies
	Mediastinal masses

teams is important for any child who may require intubation or ENT care. Treatment with oxygen, humidification, nebulized adrenaline, antibiotics and steroids is started as appropriate. Monitoring of the child is by noting degree of stridor, respiratory rate, heart rate, use of accessory movements, sternal recession, alertness and oxygen saturation. A portable chest X-ray is useful when there is a possibility of foreign body inhalation. When the clinical status of the child deteriorates to the point that intubation is required, this is best carried out within the operating department. The transfer of the child and subsequent care requires a senior clinician. The child should be breathing high-inspired oxygen, kept calm and allowed to adopt a comfortable position. Consideration should be given to administering heliox (mixtures of 21–30% oxygen and 70–79% helium) because the low density of heliox decreases resistance to turbulent airflow. Parents may accompany the child to theatre to avoid the distress of separation.

An airway strategy should be pre-formulated by senior ENT and anaesthetic staff, and equipment should be available to perform a cricothyroidotomy or rapid tracheostomy if necessary. Generally, the primary plan is to establish a surgical plane of anaesthesia with an inhalational agent. Inhalational induction using sevoflurane or halothane in oxygen is started but induction can be slow because of the combined effects of airway obstruction and ventilation–perfusion mismatch caused by atelectasis. Spontaneous respiration should be preserved at all times and CPAP is usually helpful in keeping

the airway open by combating dynamic compression and preventing atelectasis. Standard monitoring is established and intravenous access is secured once anaesthesia has been induced. Direct laryngoscopy is attempted only when the child is deeply anaesthetized, as judged by respiratory pattern, pupil size and elapsed time. Various sizes of endotracheal tubes should be ready, as often a smaller size tube may have to be used. Muscle relaxants should not be used until the airway is secure. If it is difficult to recognize the glottis on direct laryngoscopy, pressure on the chest may force some identifying bubbles to emerge.

Management of the difficult intubation scenario

There are a number of causes of difficult direct laryngoscopy, and some are associated with certain syndromes (Table 16.2). Generally, children will not tolerate an awake intubation and hence intubation is carried out under general anaesthesia. Management of the predicted difficult direct laryngoscopy is detailed below.

Preparation

Atropine can be given preoperatively either orally or intramuscularly in a dose of $20\,\mu g\,kg^{-1}$ to dry secretions. The use of sedative drugs to produce anxiolysis should be balanced against the risk of exacerbating airway obstruction and should be used with extreme caution.

Table 16.2 Causes of difficult intubation in paediatric practice

- Craniofacial syndromes
  - Pierre–Robin syndrome
  - Treacher–Collins syndrome
  - Goldenhar syndrome
- Lysosomal enzyme defects
  - Mucopolysaccharidoses/mucolipidoses
- Soft tissue swelling
  - Lymphangiomas, haemangiomas
- Others (e.g. infective, trauma, burns)

Induction of anaesthesia

Maintenance of spontaneous ventilation is paramount and an inhalation induction using either sevoflurane or halothane in 100% oxygen is the technique of choice. The aim is to attain a deep enough plane of anaesthesia to allow laryngoscopy. Obstruction to the airway during induction can be managed by change of patient position (into the lateral or even semi-prone position), and/or the use of nasal or oropharyngeal airways. Should the patient become apnoeic during the induction it is important to try to avoid assisting ventilation. Application of CPAP at this time will usually maintain oxygenation until spontaneous respiration resumes. The use of a laryngeal mask airway will often clear an obstructed airway and is a most valuable aid. Muscle relaxants should be avoided before the airway is secure to avoid the potentially disastrous 'can't ventilate, can't intubate' scenario.

Conventional techniques to aid intubation include the use of bougies and stylets which are available in paediatric sizes. The McCoy laryngoscope can also be useful. For many of these cases, however, fibreoptic intubation is necessary.

Fibreoptic intubation techniques

Two types of fibreoptic bronchoscope are available – bronchoscopes with a suction channel or ultrathin bronchoscopes without a suction channel. Bronchoscopes with a suction channel have an outer diameter of 3.5–4 mm and a tracheal tube as small as 4–4.5 mm can be railroaded over them. Ultra-thin bronchoscopes are suitable for use in neonates and infants. They have an outer diameter of approximately 2.2 mm so that a 2.5-mm tracheal tube can be railroaded over them. However, the absence of a suction channel to clear secretions is a disadvantage of these ultra-thin instruments, which can also be difficult to direct on account of their 'whippy' nature. They are easily damaged. There are two requirements for successful fibreoptic intubation in children. Firstly, one must maintain good oxygenation and deep anaesthesia to allow time to visualize the airway. Secondly, one must pre-plan the technique for placing the tracheal tube into the trachea.

Nasal or oral route

The nasal route is reserved for patients with temporo-mandibular joint problems and limited mouth opening. Bleeding caused either by the fibreoptic scope or tracheal tube can create problems. Maintenance of anaesthesia can be achieved with a nasal airway in the other nostril connected to the breathing circuit. The oral route avoids potential nasal bleeding but the angles to the larynx are more acute. Anaesthesia can be maintained via a nasal airway or a specially adapted face mask. The laryngeal mask airway, however, is now the most commonly used device to maintain anaesthesia and act as a conduit for fibreoptic intubation.

Fibreoptic intubation through a laryngeal mask airway

The laryngeal mask airway is first inserted with the patient is breathing spontaneously. Once the patient is in a deep enough plane of anaesthesia, a fibreoptic bronchoscope is introduced into the laryngeal mask airway until a view of the cords is obtained. Topical lignocaine is then sprayed onto the larynx via the suction channel and the bronchoscope is inserted into the trachea and the carina visualized. There are then a number of ways to accomplish tracheal intubation.

Railroading over the bronchoscope

An appropriate tube is loaded onto the fibrescope and railroaded into the trachea. This can be facilitated

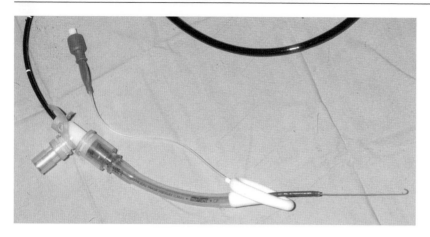

Figure 16.3 The use of a guidewire in a 'through laryngeal mask airway (LMA) intubation' technique.

by placing a second tube onto the bronchoscope (above the first) and using this as a 'pusher' to make certain that the selected tube is fully in position and not displaced on removing the laryngeal mask. The choice of the tracheal tube is also critical as choosing too big a tube will result in failure to intubate the trachea and necessitate repeating the whole procedure with a smaller tube.

Using a guidewire and airway exchange catheter

A long J-tipped guidewire is inserted via the suction channel into the trachea and the fibreoptic scope carefully removed (Figure 16.3). If the fibreoptic scope is too big for the child's trachea, the scope can sit above the cords and the guidewire inserted through the cords under direct vision. Following the removal of the bronchoscope a 'stiffening' device, such as the Cook airway exchange catheter (Cook UK Ltd, Letchworth, England), is then railroaded over the guidewire through the laryngeal mask airway. Once in place, the guidewire is removed and the position of the airway exchange catheter verified by capnography. Only when correct placement of the exchange catheter has been confirmed is the laryngeal mask airway removed. A tracheal tube can then be railroaded over the catheter. The advantages of this technique are that it can be used in children of any age, suction is available during the initial bronchoscopy and following insertion of the stiffening device the choice of the tracheal tube is less critical as it can easily be changed.

Using an airway exchange catheter without a guidewire

An ultra-thin fibreoptic bronchoscope is lubricated with saline and a Cook airway exchange catheter is fitted over it. The loaded bronchoscope is passed through the larynx and the airway exchange catheter is advanced under direct vision into the trachea. The laryngeal mask airway is then removed and a tracheal tube railroaded over the catheter into the trachea. This may be preferable to preloading an endotracheal tube as the airway exchange catheter will pass more easily into the trachea.

Key points

- There are important anatomical and physiological differences in the airway of infants and small children.
- Uncuffed tracheal tubes are usual in paediatric practice.
- The maintenance of spontaneous respiration is essential in the management of the child with stridor or difficult intubation.
- The laryngeal mask has an important role in the management of the difficult paediatric airway.
- Fibreoptic intubation techniques in paediatric practice require careful planning.
- All equipment must be immediately available.

Further reading

James I. Cuffed tubes in children. Editorial. *Paediatr Anaesth* 2001; **11**: 259–263.

Katz J, Steward DJ. *Anesthesia and Uncommon Pediatric Diseases*, 2nd edition. Philadelphia: WB Saunders, 1993.

Myer CM, Cotton RT. *The Pediatric Airway: An Interdisciplinary Approach*. Lippincott: Williams and Wilkins, 1994.

Thomas PB, Parry MG. The difficult paediatric airway: a new method of fibreoptic intubation using the laryngeal mask airway, Cook airway exchange catheter and tracheal intubation fibrescope. *Paediatr Anaesth* 2001; 11: 618–621.

Walker RWM. The laryngeal mask airway in the difficult airway: an assessment of positioning and use in fibreoptic intubation. *Paediatr Anaesth* 2000; 10: 53–58.

P.J.H. Venn

Worldwide, obstructive sleep apnoea (OSA) is the most common medical disorder affecting sleep, afflicting about 5% of the middle aged in the UK and about 80% of those affected are male. The full range of sleep disorders has been classified by the American Sleep Disorders Association (Table 17.1). The high prevalence of OSA means that anaesthetists are frequently involved with such patients presenting

either for surgery as part of treatment for the condition itself or for unrelated surgery. This chapter deals with the pathophysiology of the condition and its presenting features, investigations and treatment. It concludes with management during the peri-operative period. Sleep apnoea in children is also considered briefly.

Definition and presentation of OSA

OSA is defined as a repetitive obstruction of the upper airway during sleep causing hypoxaemia with arterial oxygen desaturation, which leads to a reduced quality of sleep. When this results in excessive daytime sleepiness (EDS), the condition is often referred to as sleep apnoea syndrome. There is almost always a history of snoring that has worsened over the preceding few years, often causing patients to sleep separately from their partners. The obstruction to the airway may arise from a number of discrete anatomical causes that are listed in Table 17.2, but in the absence of abnormal anatomy, it is relaxation of the pharyngeal constrictor muscles during sleep that allows collapse of the airway. There is evidence that these muscles are hypertonic during wakefulness, and that fatigue may become unmasked during sleep leading to excessive relaxation. Physical associations with OSA include being male, a collar size of 17 in. or greater, a large tongue and often some degree of retrognathia. The association with a high body mass index (BMI) means that most of these patients will fall into the category of potentially difficult intubations as classified in the anaesthetic literature. Medical associations include hypothyroidism, acromegaly and glycogen storage diseases, while

Table 17.1 Classification outline of sleep disorders published by the American Academy of Sleep Medicine

1 *Dyssomnias*
   A Intrinsic sleep disorders
   B Extrinsic sleep disorders
   C Circadian rhythm sleep disorders

2 *Parasomnias*
   A Arousal disorders
   B Sleep–wake transition disorders
   C Parasomnias usually associated with rapid eye movement sleep
   D Other parasomnias

3 *Medical/psychiatric sleep disorders*
   A Associated with mental disorders
   B Associated with neurological disorders
   C Associated with other medical disorders

1A *Intrinsic sleep disorders*
1   Psychophysiological insomnia
2   Sleep state misperception
3   Idiopathic insomnia
4   Narcolepsy
5   Recurrent hypersomnia
6   Idiopathic hypersomnia
7   Post-traumatic hypersomnia
8   OSA syndrome
9   Central sleep apnoea syndrome
10 Central alveolar hypoventilation syndrome
11 Periodic limb movement disorder
12 Restless legs syndrome

congenital causes include Down's syndrome, Pierre–Robin sequence and other facial anomalies. Acute nasal obstruction, such as nasal packing, can induce sleep apnoea in normal subjects and markedly worsen already affected patients.

To meet the criteria for diagnosis, apnoea from complete obstruction of the airway should occur repeatedly during sleep for more than 10 s in the presence of continued movement of the diaphragm, leading to a reduction of greater than 4% in arterial oxygen saturation (SaO_2) from the baseline. Cessation of diaphragm movement resulting in absence of ventilation is called central sleep apnoea, and, while not uncommon, is not the subject of this article. Typically in OSA, airway obstruction occurs at the level of the pharynx, hypopharynx or both for between 30 s and 1 min (and occasionally considerably longer), during which time attempted inspiration becomes increasingly vigorous as arterial oxygen desaturation progresses, finally leading to a partial arousal from sleep and sudden reopening of the airway. This causes an explosive intake of breath usually accompanied by some movement of the body or twitching of the limbs indicating sleep disruption or fragmentation. Hyperventilation follows for a short time, but as sleep deepens again, airway obstruction returns causing the cycle to restart. The worst cases may have up to 60 of these cycles per hour (apnoea index) giving 400–500 episodes in a sleep period of 8 h, with each dip in oxygen saturation as low as 60%.

This fragmented poor quality sleep leads to a lack of refreshment on awakening with EDS as measured by the Epworth Sleepiness Scale (Table 17.3). Epworth Scores above 8 out of the maximum 24 possible are regarded as above normal, and a score of greater than 12 impacts upon social and family life as well as day-time performance – particularly driving ability. Sufferers are consequently a potential danger to themselves and to others who may be dependent upon their judgement. Drivers of large goods vehicles are predisposed to the condition, partly as a result of their typical lifestyle. Although complete and repeated apnoea represents the worse case scenario, some individuals experience only partial degrees of upper airway obstruction that does not lead to overt arterial oxygen desaturation. Sleep arousals may still occur, probably due to the increased upper airway resistance causing a rise in diaphragmatic work. The resulting reduction in tidal volume due to partial upper airway obstruction is called hypopnoea, and often results in EDS in the absence of actual OSA. Recurrent night-time hypoxaemia can lead to several cardiovascular complications including arterial and pulmonary hypertension, cor pulmonale, an increased incidence of heart disease and cerebrovascular events. There is unequivocal evidence that treating OSA reduces raised arterial blood pressure.

Table 17.2 Anatomical and physiological reasons for the development of sleep disordered breathing

1 Macroglossia and a wide-tongue base
2 Retrognathia
3 Tumours of the upper airway
4 Craniofacial disorders
5 Neuromuscular disorders
6 Tonsillar hypertrophy
7 Neck girth of 17 in. or more

Table 17.3 The Epworth Sleepiness Scale

How likely are you to fall asleep or doze in the situations described below, in contrast to just feeling tired?

Use the following scale to choose the most appropriate number for each situation:

Not at all	Score 0
Slight chance	Score 1
Moderate chance	Score 2
High chance	Score 3

Activity	Score

- Sitting and reading
- Watching TV
- Sitting inactive in a public place (e.g. in a theatre or meeting)
- Sitting quietly after lunch without alcohol
- Sitting in a car as a passenger for an hour without a break
- Lying down to rest in the afternoon when circumstances permit
- Talking to someone
- In a car, while stopped for a few minutes in traffic

Clinical presentation

History

The symptoms of snoring, apnoea and EDS usually lead to consultations with ear, nose and throat (ENT) surgeons, but other medical complications may precipitate alternative presentations to chest physicians, neurologists or cardiologists. Furthermore, day-time sleepiness can mimic clinical depression and lead to psychiatric referral.

Although the clinical presentation varies and diagnosis requires an index of suspicion, the typical patient is male, with weight gain over adulthood leading to a current BMI of $30 \, \mathrm{kg \, m^{-2}}$ or more and an increase in collar size of 1.5 in. to around 17 in. during adulthood (Figure 17.1). There is a history of increasingly intrusive snoring in all positions during sleep with reports of sleep apnoea and day-time sleepiness. A full medical history should include details of the presenting complaint, as well as enquiry about nocturia, loss of libido, nightmares and sudden awakening in the night with fear, all of which are associated. Gastro-oesophageal reflux is common in this group and also leads to sudden awakening during sleep with choking and dyspnoea. A detailed cardiovascular history including the pathological consequences of hypertension should be sought, as well as prescribed and non-prescribed drugs, tobacco and alcohol consumption. More often than not, patients are already taking antihypertensive drugs, and increasing numbers are on hypocholesterolaemics and aspirin. Unfortunately, some patients present on night sedatives, their morning lack of refreshment being attributed to insomnia. Benzodiazepines, particularly, tend to worsen pharyngeal relaxation and exacerbate the situation. A commonly associated feature is poor subjective ability to breathe through the nose, and previous nasal surgery may already have been carried out, or become necessary as part of the on-going management of the condition.

Examination

A full examination of the upper airway should be undertaken, with attention to the collar size, Mallampati class, dental occlusion and pharyngeal volume. Tonsillar hypertrophy should be recorded because this may be the underlying problem, and usually is so in children presenting with OSA. The facial profile should be studied to detect degrees of retrognathia. The tongue may have crenellations at the side – small indentations on the lateral borders made by the teeth, which indicate that it is being squeezed inwards and backwards into the pharyngeal space when the mouth is closed (Figure 17.2). The pharyngeal volume is often very reduced with redundant mucosal folds limiting the lateral diameter (Figure 17.3). It is also useful to ask the patient to sublux the jaw forwards to measure the amount of movement, because good degrees of movement

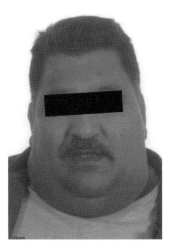

Figure 17.1 The typical facial features of a patient with OSA. Notice the width of the neck.

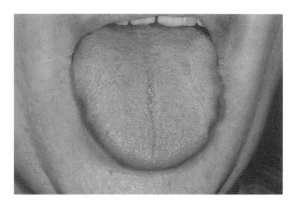

Figure 17.2 The typical appearance of the tongue in a patient with OSA. Notice the 'crenellations' (indentations) on the lateral borders of the tongue made by the teeth and the Mallampati score of 4.

of greater than 5 mm may allow treatment with intra-oral mandibular advancement devices rather than continuous positive airway pressure (CPAP) devices.

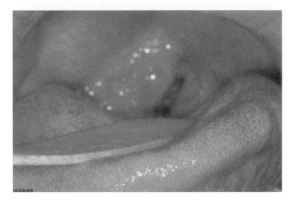

Figure 17.3 The restricted pharyngeal volume with redundant mucosal folds often seen in association with OSA.

Investigations

Investigations include blood tests to exclude other causes of EDS, such as hypothyroidism and narcolepsy, but the diagnosis is readily confirmed by carrying out a sleep study called a polysomnogram (PSG). Full polysomnography includes monitoring of the chest movement, airflow dynamics, heart rate and blood pressure, SaO_2 and the electroencephalogram (EEG), all during sleep. EEG monitoring is used to assess the stages of sleep (Stages I–IV non-rapid eye movement (REM) or REM sleep) and is a valuable tool in the diagnosis of complex sleep disorders. However, at least in the UK, comparatively few sleep laboratories have this facility, and cardiorespiratory monitoring alone is usually carried out; this being adequate to diagnose OSA. Video telemetry using an infrared camera for night-time recording combined with sound is a very useful

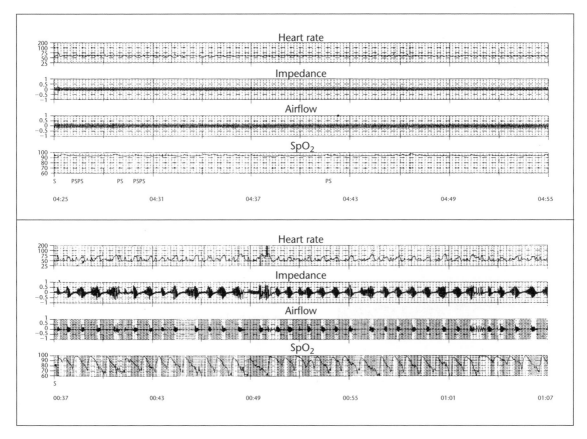

Figure 17.4 Respiratory traces recorded for half an hour from two subjects while asleep. The four channels from top to bottom show heart rate, chest movement, airflow and SaO_2. The top trace is taken during unobstructed quiet sleep and shows a steady heart rate with normal respiration and levels of oxygen saturation. The lower trace shows OSA with cyclical dips in oxygen saturation due to regular cessation of airflow with consequent rises and falls in heart rate as each partial arousal from sleep occurs.

supplement. Comparisons of a normal respiratory PSG with one from a patient with florid OSA are shown in Figure 17.4.

Treatment of OSA

The gold standard of treatment for OSA is to submit the patient to nasal CPAP (nCPAP) while asleep. CPAP devices are now in common usage worldwide, and a wide range of products is available. CPAP is applied to the airway through a nasal mask (Figure 17.5), and works by applying positive airway pressure to the pharynx throughout the breathing cycle to overcome the obstructive forces due to pharyngeal collapse. CPAP is usually commenced in hospital for one night under supervision while the correct level of airway pressure measured in centimetres of H_2O is set for the individual. While the pressure energy should be high enough to overcome the pharyngeal collapse causing the obstruction, it should not be so high as to reach the lower airway and raise the functional residual capacity, because there is evidence that this in itself disrupts

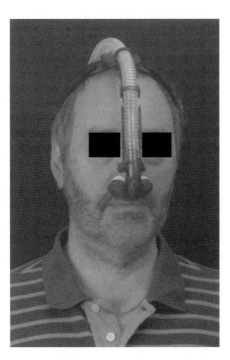

Figure 17.5 Application of nCPAP to the airway using nasal prongs and harness. The minimal amount of hardware attached to the patient's face increases the acceptability of the device.

sleep. Pressure requirements range from as low as $5 \, cmH_2O$ to as high as $15–20 \, cmH_2O$ depending upon the severity of the obstruction.

Many studies have been carried out to evaluate and predict the compliance to treatment of patients who use CPAP at home. Clearly, non-compliance brings no benefit or relief from symptoms, but every laboratory has its group of such patients. Good compliance predictors include self-referral due to EDS (as opposed to referral due to snoring under pressure from partners or family), a patent nasal airway, and most importantly, relief of day-time sleepiness on nCPAP with an improved quality of life. Despite treating OSA adequately with CPAP, about 10% of patients remain excessively sleepy by day, and the reason for this has recently been debated but remains undecided. The level of compliance is recorded in hours of usage by a meter built into the device, and at least 4 h of use per night is necessary for a reduction in EDS as evaluated by pre- and post-treatment Epworth Scores.

There are no serious side effects of nCPAP treatment, but minor side effects may decrease compliance and benefit. Of these, inflammation of the nasal mucosa from the pressurized airflow often leads to symptoms of rhinitis and nasal blockage that can be troublesome during early treatment, and is sometimes a reason for failure of compliance. Nasal blockage usually causes the user to mouth breathe with loss of pharyngeal pressure, causing airflow entering through the nose to escape through the mouth. Such patients awaken with sore and dry throats that may be distressing. Nasal blockage can be treated with topical steroid sprays, but responds better to humidification of the pressurized airflow, the humidifier being either an integral part of the machine design, or attached to it (Figure 17.6). Where the nasal airway persistently blocks despite simple measures, a full face mask covering the nose and mouth may be helpful, with resort to nasal surgery if all else fails. Other problems of using nCPAP include noise emission from the device disturbing the sleep of the partner or patient, discomfort from the mask and feelings of claustrophobia.

While the most noticeable effect of nCPAP is to reduce day-time sleepiness, physiological benefits also occur. Hypertensive patients treated with

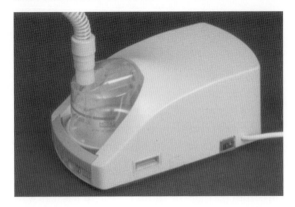

Figure 17.6 The Fisher Pakel CPAP device with an inbuilt heated water bath for humidification of inspired air.

nCPAP show a beneficial reduction in both systolic and diastolic blood pressure, the effect of which appears to increase with time. The strong association of asthma with OSA also benefits, as does nocturia, the reduction of which improves sleep quality in itself. With time, patients become very adept in managing their nCPAP therapy, putting it on, adjusting it and going to sleep within only a few minutes.

As previously stated, some patients can be treated for mild OSA with mandibular advancement devices, which posture the mandible forwards pulling the tongue away from the posterior pharyngeal wall via the suprahyoid muscles. Mandibular advancement depends upon a partial dislocation of the temporomandibular joint. Patients who benefit most from this treatment tend to be retrognathic with a class II dental malocclusion, where the bottom incisors lie behind the top incisors when the mouth is closed. They have snoring predominantly from behind the tongue that may cause varying degrees of upper airway obstruction during sleep, even in the absence of true OSA. More recently, radio frequency coagulation of the palate (somnoplasty) and ablation of the base of the tongue have been used with some success in the treatment of palatal snoring, having replaced the unpleasant operation of uvulopalatopharyngoplasty (UPPP). There is no place for UPPP in the modern management of sleep apnoea, although laser-assisted palatoplasty is still carried out on the unwary and many patients present to sleep clinics with OSA who have previously undergone such

surgery. Post-operative infection and the later and more serious complication of velopharyngeal incompetence combined with poor results have led to a sharp decline in its use.

OSA and anaesthesia

Pre-operative assessment

The most serious risk for patients with OSA undergoing surgery is loss of the airway caused by the use of anaesthetic, sedative and opioid drugs, combined with the increased risk of anaesthesia from clinical obesity and hypertension. The high prevalence of OSA means that anaesthetists will meet it frequently. Most sufferers remain undiagnosed, and reliance cannot, therefore, be put on the patient to volunteer information about their symptoms. Patients may present for surgery as part of the overall management of their sleep apnoea, most often on the nasal airway, palate, tongue or tonsils, where there is the added complication of shared airway anaesthesia. However, the undiagnosed patient presenting for unrelated surgery poses the greatest risk and, where there is a suspicion of sleep apnoea, elective surgery should be postponed until the patient has been fully investigated and treated.

Planning for surgery should start well before the day of admission, because special investigations may be needed as part of the peri-operative workup. Previous anaesthetic records grading ease of direct laryngoscopy and intubation are invaluable if available. All patients using CPAP at home should be instructed to bring their device with them on the day of admission for use during their hospital stay, and the staff looking after them on the ward and in the recovery room should be familiar with CPAP and its use.

The anaesthetic assessment of the airway should begin routinely by enquiring about a history of snoring or apnoea during sleep. Most patients will be aware of the disharmony in the bedroom due to their condition even if no medical help has previously been sought. A concurrent history of day-time sleepiness suggests some degree of airway obstruction during sleep that may well be transposed to anaesthesia. Enquiry about cardiorespiratory symptoms is mandatory to evaluate right and left ventricular function and the presence of cor pulmonale, together with the consequences of end organ dysfunction. Examination and prediction of the difficult airway has been extensively documented in the anaesthetic literature, and a detailed analysis will not be given here. However, the degree of mouth opening, Mallampati score and thyromental distance should be recorded, together with a Wilson summation score.

A frank discussion with the patient is necessary about the increased risk of general anaesthesia and should include a detailed explanation of the anaesthetic technique deemed appropriate. The high association with clinical obesity and acid reflux may affect the planning of the anaesthetic.

Pre-medication with sedatives and opioids should be avoided or used with extreme caution if deemed absolutely necessary. Constant vigilance is required once these drugs have been administered, and monitoring of the SaO_2 should be considered.

Anaesthetic technique

Although this group of patients present a formidable challenge to the anaesthetist in terms of intubation, extubation and post-operative analgesia, the literature on anaesthetic management is sparse. Of interest is a recent retrospective study that concludes that while morbid obesity in itself is not a predictor of difficult direct laryngoscopy, a history of OSA is so, with Cormack grades III and IV views in 90% of OSA patients studied.

No global rules can be applied to the choice of anaesthetic technique, and each patient should be considered according to their individual needs. However, induction under full monitoring is required, and whatever means is used to secure the airway most agree that tracheal intubation is preferable to use of the laryngeal mask airway. Regard should be given to possible regurgitation of stomach acid during induction. A full range of aids for difficult intubation should be ready, and attendant staff should be familiar with the use of such equipment. Some authors advocate awake fibre-optic intubation under topical

anaesthesia for all patients with OSA, although obtunded airway reflexes after local anaesthesia to the upper airway has been reported to cause increased levels of obstruction in the post-operative period. Whatever technique is chosen for induction and intubation, the attention and skill of all staff are of paramount importance, and at least two plans should be made to maintain the airway in the event of failure of the first. Extubation should be predicted to be 'stormy' and not be undertaken until the patient is awake. Intra-operative use of local anaesthesia for pain relief will allow sparing administration of opioid drugs, and regional techniques using infusions are useful adjuncts in the post-operative period.

Although avoidance of sedative and opioid drugs during the peri-operative period is the recommended practice, sedatives and opioids have reportedly been used freely in conjunction with CPAP therapy without complication in the post-operative period.

Post-operative management

The patient's CPAP device should be sent to the recovery room during surgery and made ready for use immediately on emergence from anaesthesia. Under no circumstances should the patient be left unattended or without cardiorespiratory monitoring until fully awake, and even then consideration should be given to the enterohepatic circulation of any sedative or opiate drugs. Up to 20% of patients require major medical intervention, including re-intubation, in the immediate post-operative period. Nursing staff should be familiar with such complications and be ready to maintain a difficult airway if needed, and the anaesthetist should obviously be immediately available. Subsequent management in an intensive care or high dependency unit should be considered for any major surgical intervention, especially vascular surgery, where significant oxygen desaturation has been recorded during the first two post-operative nights, possibly due to rebound levels of REM sleep following anaesthesia. Patients with known or suspected lesser degrees of OSA should be prescribed nocturnal oxygen post-operatively and for at least one night after opioid therapy has stopped. Oxygen does not prevent airway obstruction, but can prevent desaturation.

Sleep apnoea in children

OSA in children is a specialized area, but most often presents on ENT operating lists for correction of adenoidal or tonsillar hypertrophy, despite a lack of evidence about the efficacy of such surgery in the literature. It is, therefore, appropriate to enquire from the parents about a history of snoring and the child's breathing quality during sleep. A diminished ventilatory response to CO_2 has been recorded in these patients and they require trained paediatric staff in the recovery room. Although children are less amenable than adults, they can be successfully managed with CPAP in specialized centres; Great Ormond Street Hospital for Sick Children in London claiming success in up to 86% of children of various ages with OSA not relieved by adenotonsillectomy. Rarer associations with OSA in children include congenital conditions, such as the mucopolysaccharidoses, Down's syndrome and hypothyroidism. Conditions of craniofacial deformity, such as Pierre–Robin sequence, Treacher-Collins syndrome and Goldenhars syndrome may be associated with OSA. Such cases require treatment in specialized centres with multidisciplinary planning and should not be managed outside an appropriate environment.

Key points

- OSA is a common condition, often unrecognized.
- OSA recognized at pre-operative evaluation needs proper assessment before surgery.
- Airway management may be more difficult, intra- and post-operatively.
- OSA increases post-operative morbidity and mortality.
- Established therapy, such as CPAP, should be continued in the post-operative period.
- Opioid therapy presents particular problems and patients require cardiorespiratory monitoring.
- Supplemental oxygen is required for one night longer than opioid therapy.

Further reading

Adenotonsillectomy for obstructive sleep apnoea in children. *Cochrane Database Syst Rev* 2003; **1**: CD003136.

Benumof JL. Obstructive sleep apnea in the adult obese patient: implications for airway management. *Anesthesiol Clin North Am* 2002; **20**: 789–811.

Biro P, Kaplan V, Bloch KE. Anesthetic management of a patient with obstructive sleep apnoea syndrome and difficult airway access. *J Clin Anaesth* 1995; **7**: 417–421.

Brown KA, Morin I, Hickey C, Manoukian JJ, Nixon GM, Brouillett RT. Urgent adenotonsillectomy: an analysis of risk factors associated with postoperative respiratory morbidity. *Anesthesiology* 2003; **99**: 586–595.

Eastwood PR, Szollosi I, Platt PR, Hillman DR. Comparison of upper airway collapse during general anaesthesia and sleep. *Lancet* 2002; **359**: 1207–1209.

Edelman NH, Santiago TV (Eds). *Breathing Disorders of Sleep.* London: Churchill Livingstone, 1986.

Ezri T, Medalion B, Weisenberg M, Szmuk P, Warters RD. Increased body mass index *per se* is not a predictor of difficult laryngoscopy. *Can J Anaesth* 2003; **30**: 179–183.

Jarrell L. Preoperative diagnosis and postoperative management of adult patients with obstructive sleep apnea syndrome: a review of the literature. *J Perianesth Nurs* 1999; **14**: 193–200.

Jones JG, Jordan C, Scudder C *et al.* Episodic postoperative oxygen desaturation: the value of added oxygen. *J Roy Soc Med* 1985; **78**: 1019–1022.

Logan AG, Tkacova R, Perlikowski SM, Leung RS *et al.* Refractory hypertension and sleep apnoea: effect of CPAP on blood pressure and baroreceptor reflex. *Eur Repir J* 2003; **21**: 241–247.

Massa F, Gonsalez S, Laverty A, Wallis C, Lane R. The use of nasal continuous positive airway pressure to treat obstructive sleep apnoea. *Arch Dis Child* 2002; **87**: 438–443.

Stradling JR. *Handbook of Sleep Related Breathing Disorders.* UK: Oxford University Press, 1993.

Strauss SG, Lynn AM, Bratton SL, Nespeca MK. Ventilatory response to CO_2 in children with obstructive sleep apnea from adenotonsillar hypertrophy. *Anesth Analg* 1999; **89**: 328–332.

Wetmore SJ, Scrima L, Hiller FC. Sleep apnea in epistaxis patients treated with nasal packs. *Otolaryngol Head Neck Surg* 1988; **98**: 596–599.

THE AIRWAY IN CERVICAL TRAUMA 18

P. Ford and D.A. Gabbott

Introduction

Acute trauma victims often require immediate tracheal intubation and when this is necessary there are a number of concurrent problems to consider. There may or may not be immediate airway obstruction caused by extensive disruption to normal airway anatomy from both blunt and penetrating injuries. Airway haematoma and oedema may be present and certain injury patterns are recognized as causing airway compromise including the 'flail' mandible, where loss of support for the tongue anteriorly encourages it to fall backwards. Additionally, there may be severe haemorrhage and other debris present in the airway, which can make fibre-optic techniques impractical. There is invariably a full stomach with the associated risk of aspiration and finally, one must always consider injuries to the cervical spine.

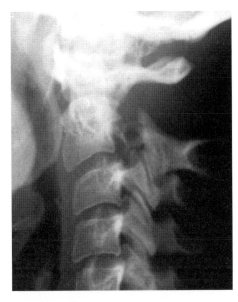

Figure 18.1 'Hangman's' fracture of C2. Patient complained of neck pain after hitting windscreen in a road traffic accident (RTA).

Cervical spine injury

Approximately, 5% of severe, blunt injuries to the head and neck have cervical spine damage. Up to 14% of these injuries may be unstable, and between 1% and 5% of these injuries are initially missed. Fractures most commonly occur at the level of C2 and dislocations at the C5/6/7 regions (Figure 18.1). All such injuries may predispose to further airway obstruction from haematoma formation and soft tissue oedema in the neck (Table 18.1). Sadly, about 5% of patients admitted to hospital with cervical spine trauma will suffer a neurological deterioration after admission. Some of these deteriorations occur for no discernible reason, but some are associated with general anaesthesia. It

seems sensible, therefore, to assume that there is an un-quantified risk of neurological deterioration in patients undergoing general anaesthesia with cervical spine injuries. In those with a confirmed, isolated cervical spine injury who are awake, co-operative and not in immediate need of emergency surgery, neck stabilization procedures can be undertaken using local anaesthesia, for example application of a halo. There is then time for the stomach to empty, and where general anaesthesia becomes necessary, the use of awake, flexible fibre-optic laryngoscopy is often the preferred method for securing the airway if tracheal intubation is required and a halo is in place. Such a technique allows neurological re-assessment prior to commencing

Table 18.1 Broken neck

Epidemiology
- Male : Female – 4 : 1
- Median age – 25 years

Of trauma admissions
- 80% have skeletal injury
- 6% have (radiological) spinal injury
- 2.6% have a spinal cord injury (SCI) (i.e. roughly 50% of fractures have an SCI)
- SCI without radiographic abnormality (SCIWORA) – especially children and the old
- 40% of cervical fracture patients have radiological vertebral artery damage
- 5% of cervical spine trauma patients deteriorate neurologically after admission
- 7% of severe head injury patients have cervical spine injury
- 40% of patients with an SCI have a head injury

surgery and even the possibility of surgical positioning before inducing general anaesthesia. Many of these patients, however, will require emergency surgery and often immediate tracheal intubation for a variety of medical problems.

'Clearing' the cervical spine in unconscious patients

This is often a practical problem in intensive care. It is believed that the combination of lateral, arterioposterior (AP) and open-mouth radiographs has a sensitivity of about 100% for bone injury, if it is possible to obtain technically satisfactory views, which is frequently difficult. Computed tomography (CT) scans should be obtained if radiographs are unsatisfactory, and since most patients will be having a cranial scan, it can actually be more convenient to obtain a CT scan than the radiographic series. Ligamentous injury cannot be excluded by radiographs or CT scans. Exclusion procedures for ligamentous injury are a matter of debate. Some advocate flexion/extension fluoroscopy, while others believe magnetic resonance imaging (MRI) scanning is the safest option. Others maintain that the risks involved in obtaining an MRI scan outweigh the small chance of an unstable ligamentous injury being present without bony injury. There is currently no consensus on the best procedure.

Direct laryngoscopy

Direct laryngoscopy is the most common method used to secure the airway in a trauma setting. It allows suction, direct visualization of the larynx and any associated airway trauma, and retrieval of any foreign material. During normal laryngoscopy, the dominant motion of the cervical spine is extension with the greatest amount of movement occurring at the atlanto-occipital and atlanto–axial joints. Without external stabilization, the amount of movement at these joints during laryngoscopy has been measured at 7–9° and 4–5°, respectively. Retrospective analysis of patients with potential cervical spine injuries has shown the technique of direct laryngoscopy to be safe; however, a few anecdotal reports of patients developing neurological deterioration following laryngoscopy and tracheal intubation have caused some to doubt the safety of the procedure. Further analysis of these cases implicating direct laryngoscopy as a possible cause of spinal cord damage has revealed little evidence that the technique was to blame as there are many confounding factors including total time of spinal cord compression and vascular compromise.

The 'gum elastic' bougie is probably the most useful adjunct to facilitate tracheal intubation during direct laryngoscopy of trauma patients. Its use in the patient with an injured cervical spine allows the anaesthetist to accept a sub-optimal view of the larynx, thereby reducing the force and by implicating the movement of the cervical spine during laryngoscopy. The ability to pass the device blindly under the epiglottis and feel for tracheal 'clicks' or achieve 'hold up' within the bronchial tree are further advantages when both time and the laryngeal view are limited. The newer disposable bougies may not prove so useful in this setting, however, as they appear to possess less 'memory'.

Choice of laryngoscope

The standard laryngoscope blade used by many anaesthetists is the Macintosh. It is curved and views of the larynx are obtained by placing the tip of the blade in the vallecula and lifting the epiglottis up and out of the way. In an attempt to reduce movement of the cervical spine, other laryngoscopes and blades have been studied. The Miller laryngoscope has a straight blade, the tip of which is passed beyond the epiglottis. The blade is then used to lift the epiglottis directly to obtain a view of the vocal cords. This has the theoretical advantage of reducing the force during laryngoscopy; however, in practice this has not been shown to reduce movement of the neck. The Bullard laryngoscope is a rigid fibre-optic laryngoscope which allows visualization of the larynx without having to align the oral, pharyngeal and tracheal axes, thereby allowing the neck to remain in the neutral position. Research has shown this laryngoscope to be superior to standard laryngoscope blades with regards to reducing cervical spine movement; however, its use is complicated by prolonged intubation times, 'fogging' and 'soiling' of the field of view and a lack of competency in the hands of many anaesthetists.

The levering laryngoscope (Figure 18.2), first described by McCoy, is a modification of the Macintosh blade with an angulated tip which can be activated during laryngoscopy. It has found a more defined role in patients with cervical spine injuries and use of this laryngoscope, with the tip in the angulated position, reduces the incidence of difficult laryngoscopy in patients whose necks are maintained in a neutral position. Thus, the levering laryngoscope may reduce the force transmitted by the anaesthetist, and thereby reduce motion of the cervical spine if difficult laryngoscopy is encountered.

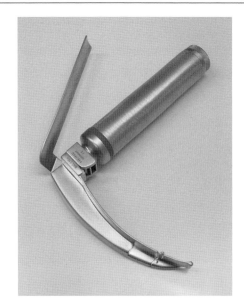

Figure 18.2 Levering laryngoscope.

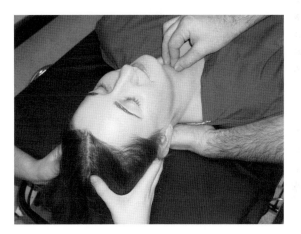

Figure 18.3 MILS and two-handed cricoid pressure.

Cricoid pressure

Tracheal intubation of acute trauma patients takes place in the presence of a full stomach and there is, therefore, a risk of aspiration during the procedure. Cricoid pressure, performed with one or two hands, aims to compress the hypopharynx, thereby reducing passive regurgitation. The technique has also been used to improve the view at laryngoscopy with pressure applied backwards, upwards and to the right (BURP). The double-handed technique produces a better view at laryngoscopy than the single-handed technique and is, therefore, the method of choice (Figure 18.3). It may also reduce any potential cervical spine movement that the single-handed technique may induce. Motion of the cervical spine during application of cricoid pressure, however, has generally been found to be minimal, and the technique, therefore, appears safe to carry out on patients with unstable cervical spines. Orogastric tubes should be left *in situ* as their presence improves the efficacy of cricoid pressure and simultaneously allows gastric venting.

There are disadvantages of applying cricoid pressure. Firstly, incorrect application can make laryngoscopy and mask ventilation more difficult. Secondly, it may make positioning of a laryngeal mask airway (LMA) or intubating LMA (ILMA) more difficult or impossible, as it reduces the capacity of the hypopharynx and prevents the distal end of such devices from sitting in their correct position. Cricoid pressure, therefore, may have to be relaxed or removed completely during their insertion.

Cervical spine immobilization

During the initial management of any trauma patient, cervical spine immobilization using one of several available methods is now a standard procedure until cervical spine injury has been excluded. It must be appreciated, however, that none of the methods available are able to restrict neck motion completely. For example, the soft collar only provides the very minimum amount of restraint and, therefore, should not be used. The application of Gardner–Wells forceps permits the least movement of the neck, but in the acute setting it is often not practical. Between these two extremes are the techniques of using a rigid cervical collar together with sand bags and tape or manual in-line stabilization (MILS) of the neck. Most patients arriving at the hospital following acute trauma will have had a rigid collar applied in the pre-hospital phase of their management. Such collars, however, make laryngoscopy more difficult, increasing the likelihood of a grade 3 or 4 view of the larynx and they should, therefore, be removed before direct laryngoscopy is performed and MILS applied. MILS will reduce cervical spine motion by up to 60% and is less likely to impair the view at laryngoscopy. It is, therefore, the preferred method of neck stabilization in the acute setting allowing the anaesthetist to apply an increased upward and forward force, which would not otherwise have been possible through fear of lifting the head and moving the neck. To apply MILS, an assistant places a hand on each side of the patient's head with the fingertips pressed on each mastoid process and the hands then pressed firmly into the trolley/spinal board.

The thumbs then firmly grasp the occiput (Figure 18.2). During laryngoscopy, the hands act to oppose any forces applied by the anaesthetist, so as to maintain a motionless cervical spine. Encouraging axial traction during MILS can produce a distraction injury to the spinal cord and should, therefore, be avoided. If tracheal intubation is proving difficult, it may become necessary to reduce the grip applied bearing in mind that some cervical spine movement may then occur. This decision has to be carefully balanced in light of the clinical condition of the patient, the degree of hypoxia and the immediate availability of other appropriate airway adjuncts and devices.

Airway adjuncts

The LMA is a well proven airway adjunct in circumstances of a failed intubation or difficult airway. It is a device that protects the airway from sources of soiling above the larynx, which in the case of trauma patients is often blood. It is no great surprise that its use has been promoted in patients with injured cervical spines. Although routine insertion involves flexion of the neck and head extension, insertion of an LMA is only marginally more difficult with the head in a neutral position. During insertion, however, the LMA can produce transient pressures in the hypopharynx of $>200\,cmH_2O$. This has the theoretical possibility of causing posterior displacement of an unstable cervical spine, although no reports of this phenomenon causing neurological deterioration have occurred thus far. If intubation of the trachea is impossible and use of an LMA is considered, regurgitation should be anticipated and suction applied since pressure to the cricoid cartilage may reduce lower oesophageal sphincter tone.

The ILMA (Figure 18.4) may have some advantages over the existing LMA in that higher airway pressures can be generated (up to $30\,cmH_2O$), intubation through the device is more successful than the conventional LMA and insertion with the neck in a neutral position appears to be easier. Again there may be concerns about the amount of

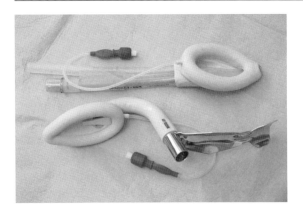

Figure 18.4 ILMA and Proseal.

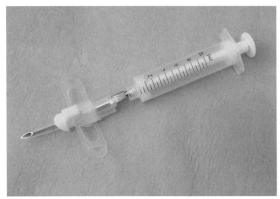

Figure 18.5 Quicktrach, VBM Medical.

force the rigid metal tube of the ILMA imparts to the cervical spine and its effectiveness in the presence of cricoid pressure is severely impaired.

The Proseal LMA (Figure 18.4) is a further modification of the LMA. The device has an additional lumen, allowing direct drainage of the oesophagus and a posterior cuff which allows ventilation at airway pressures in excess of $30 \, cmH_2O$. A recent study has shown it to be easier to insert than the LMA in patients with MILS applied.

A variety of other supraglottic airway devices are now available. Few of these have been evaluated in the trauma setting, however, other than the Combitube. This double-lumen, double-cuff device is passed blindly into the mouth and pharynx. It allows ventilation of the patient's lungs, whether the tube enters the oesophagus or trachea, although placement is nearly always in the oesophagus. The Combitube has some distinct advantages over other available airway adjuncts. It occludes the oesophagus with a distal cuff and like the Proseal LMA allows 'venting' of oesophageal and gastric contents via one of the two lumens. High airway pressures can be generated (up to $30 \, cmH_2O$) and it can be inserted with the neck in a neutral position making it useful in victims of trauma. Insertion of the device while wearing a hard cervical collar, however, is clinically very difficult, probably as a result of its size and poor mouth opening. Many studies have also highlighted problems with the Combitube. It may be difficult to insert without correct training

and it can cause pharyngeal or laryngeal trauma during insertion.

Cricothyrotomy

If laryngoscopy fails and the above airway adjuncts also fail to provide adequate ventilation and oxygenation then the patient will inevitably perish unless access to the trachea is secured in an efficient manner. This 'can't intubate, can't ventilate' scenario necessitates creating an entry point into the airway somewhere below the larynx. In patients who have severely disrupted upper airway anatomy, this should be performed early in the course of managing this situation.

Anatomically, the cricothyroid membrane provides the most suitable landmark. The membrane is relatively avascular with the exception of the superiorly positioned cricothyroid artery. It is easily accessible, demanding less neck extension than that required for tracheostomy and is protected posteriorly by the cricoid cartilage. A variety of cricothyrotomy techniques can be taught including the use of a needle and small bore cannula, a larger bore, purposely designed trocar and cannula (Figure 18.5) and a more formal surgical airway involving insertion of a tracheal tube. Each of these techniques has its merits and demerits. The needle and cannula technique requires a high-pressure oxygen source and the formal surgical airway has the most complications. Some motion of the unstable cervical spine during performance of a surgical cricothyrotomy has also been shown to occur with 1–2 mm of AP motion and up to 1 mm of axial compression. The greatest amount of motion occurs during insertion of the tracheal tube due to downward pressure of the stabilizing hand. Whichever technique is chosen, cricothyrotomy is a life-saving procedure and small amounts of cervical spine motion under these circumstances must be considered acceptable risks.

When used appropriately, survival from cricothyrotomy is encouraging. Training is of paramount importance if the procedure is to be performed efficiently and with confidence in times of crisis. Mannequins are available and animal tissue preparations are realistic teaching aides. The best training is provided by using cadavers. Finally, if we are to encourage use of this technique, we should make the equipment readily available at sites where it is most likely to be used, and ensure that it is not only utilized as a technique of 'last resort' in the moribund patient.

Conclusion

In a recent review of airway management after upper cervical spine injury, Crosby concluded that airway procedures producing neck movement represent little risk to underlying neural elements if such movement is within physiologically normal limits. Furthermore, he concluded that there is no data suggesting better outcomes with any particular airway management technique. Prudent, cautious care and maintenance of spinal immobilization are important factors in limiting the risk of secondary neurological injury and while all airway manoeuvres result in some degree of neck movement, this is small and reduced significantly by MILS.

The article recently published by Dunhan et al. (2003) from the Eastern Association for the Surgery of Trauma recommends tracheal intubation for any trauma patients who have airway obstruction, hypoventilation, severe hypoxaemia, Glasgow coma scale (GCS) < 8 and severe haemorrhagic shock. Currently, a rapid sequence induction (RSI) of anaesthesia with two-handed cricoid pressure,

suction and MILS of the neck is the recommended technique for intubation. Pre-oxygenation may be difficult and oxygenation after induction of anaesthesia, using gentle positive pressure ventilation in the presence of cricoid pressure, may be the only way that the oxygen saturation can be optimized prior to attempting oral tracheal intubation. A bougie and levering laryngoscope should be available as well as back-up suction to clear a severely soiled airway if the first suction unit fails at a critical moment. If laryngoscopy is proving difficult the generation of 'air bubbles', by pressing on the patient's chest, may allow identification of laryngeal structures and the subsequent passage of a bougie. If intubation fails, then an appropriate supraglottic airway device should be inserted and if this proves futile then a cricothyrotomy should be performed.

Key points

- A small number of patients deteriorate neurologically after admission with cervical spine injury.
- Direct laryngoscopy is believed to be safe so long as cervical spine immobilization is applied.
- No method of immobilization keeps the cervical spine completely motionless.
- Remove rigid collars, sand bags and tape prior to attempting oral tracheal intubation and use MILS.
- Have a low threshold for using the gum elastic bougie and levering laryngoscope.
- In the 'can't intubate, can't ventilate' situation perform a cricothyrotomy.

Further reading

Criswell JC, Parr MJ, Nolan JP. Emergency airway management in patients with cervical spine injuries. *Anaesthesia* 1994; **49**: 900–903.

Crosby E. Airway management after upper cervical spine injury: what have we learned? *Can J Anaesth* 2002; **49**: 733–744.

Crosby ET, Lui A. The adult cervical spine: implications for airway management. *Can J Anaesth* 1990; **37**: 77–93.

Donaldson III WF, Heil BV, Donaldson VP *et al.* The effect of airway maneuvers on the unstable C1–C2 segment. A cadaver study. *Spine* 1997; **22**: 1215–1218.

Dunham CM, Barraco RD, Clark DE, Daley BJ, Davis III FE, Gibbs MA, Knuth T, Letarte PB, Luchette FA, Omert L, Weireter LJ, Wiles III CE, EAST Practice Management Guidelines Work Group. Guidelines for emergency tracheal intubation immediately after traumatic injury. *J Trauma* 2003; **55**: 162–179.

Gabbott DA. Laryngoscopy using the McCoy laryngoscope after application of a cervical collar. *Anaesthesia* 1996; **51**: 808–811.

Gerling MC, Davis DP, Hamilton RS *et al.* Effect of surgical cricothyrotomy on the unstable cervical spine in a cadaver model of intubation. *J Emerg Med* 2001; **20(1)**: 1–5.

Lennarson PJ, Smith D, Todd MM *et al.* Segmental cervical spine motion during orotracheal intubation of the intact and injured spine with and without external stabilization. *J Neurosurg* 2000; **92**: 201–206.

McLeod AD, Calder I. Spinal cord injury and direct laryngoscopy – the legend lives on. *Br J Anaesth* 2000; **84**: 705–709.

Mercer M, Gabbott DA. Insertion of the Combitube airway with the cervical spine immobilized in a rigid cervical collar. *Anaesthesia* 1998; **53**: 971–974.

Nolan JP, Wilson ME. Orotracheal intubation in patients with potential cervical spine injuries. An indication for the gum elastic bougie. *Anaesthesia* 1993; **48**: 630–633.

I. Calder

Difficulty with the airway and cervical spine disease are associated because adequate flexion/extension movement at the cranio-cervical junction is an essential requirement of airway management.

The three main problems are as follows:

1 Difficult direct laryngoscopy.
2 Post-operative airway obstruction.
3 Spinal cord damage.

Difficult direct laryngoscopy

This is common when the occipito-atlanto-axial complex is involved by disease. Osteoarthritis/cervical spondylosis can involve the upper two cervical vertebrae and their joints, but top end disease is most often due to rheumatoid arthritis, tumours and iatrogenic interventions (fixation devices) (Figures 19.1 and 19.2).

Poor mouth opening is common in cervical disease. There is an association between cervical arthritides, especially rheumatoid and temporo-mandibular joint (TMJ) disease. Impaired cranio-cervical extension has been shown to prevent full mouth opening. The mechanism is uncertain.

Grade 3 laryngoscopy occurs in about 7% of patients with cervical spondylosis, but the prevalence can be over 40% in patients having surgery for cervical rheumatoid arthritis.

Post-operative airway obstruction

The reported incidence of this has been as high as 6%, with re-intubation being required in 2%. The

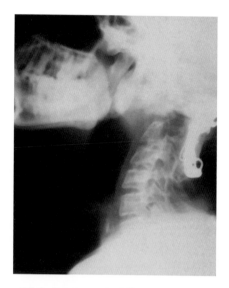

Figure 19.1 Cranio-cervical fixator in place. Difficult laryngoscopy is likely.

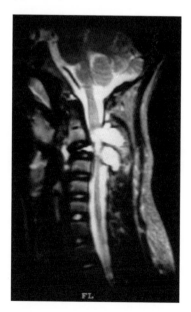

Figure 19.2 Tumour in C3, C5 and T1. Cranio-cervical junction unaffected – difficult laryngoscopy unlikely.

classic cause is a haematoma in the wound after anterior cervical surgery. However, the haematoma may be small, or even absent. The problem seems to be due to interference with venous and lymphatic drainage, and it is commoner after long operations. Airway obstruction due to tissue swelling is a particular problem after front and back surgery, where a patient has anterior surgery followed by posterior surgery in the prone position. Airway obstruction after cervical surgery is sometimes neglected because of misunderstandings about symptoms and signs.

Symptoms and signs of post-operative airway obstruction after anterior cervical surgery

---

1 These patients typically *do not* have stridor.
2 They complain of *'not being able to breathe'*, want to sit up and are anxious.
3 Arterial oxygen saturation (S_aO_2) is *not* a reliable guide. Saturation may remain normal (particularly if extra oxygen is being applied) until obstruction is virtually complete.
4 The presence of a drain *does not* affect the incidence of obstruction. In many cases no haematoma is present, and the problem is tissue oedema.

Management

a *Give oxygen and open the wound*: Evacuate any haematoma. Relieving tissue compression and lymphatic/venous obstruction by opening the wound may be enough to avert disaster – in one report (where the neck had become swollen due to fluid leaking from shoulder arthroscopy irrigation) the skin incision made to perform emergency tracheostomy relieved obstruction. The patient should be removed to intensive therapy unit (ITU)/high dependency unit (HDU) and observed.

b *The decision to re-intubate should be based on the patient's symptoms*: Re-intubate if the patient is distressed. Tracheal intubation is often very difficult, due to folds of swollen pharyngeal mucosa. A *gum elastic bougie* has often been the difference between success and failure. A laryngeal mask airway (LMA) may relieve the obstruction, but tracheal intubation should be performed – the glottis seems to become swollen less quickly than the looser paraglottic tissue.

c The tracheal tube should be left in place for about 12–24 h.

Spinal cord damage

Patients do (fortunately rarely) suffer spinal cord damage during general anaesthesia. The causation is uncertain. Airway management is a possible cause, but seems an unlikely one, because:

a There is little movement of the cervical vertebrae at direct laryngoscopy or LMA insertion – even in cadaver preparations of C0/1/2/3 rendered experimentally unstable.
b Direct laryngoscopy is a short procedure. Experimental spinal cord injury studies have demonstrated that if small deformations of the cord are produced, lengthy periods of time are required to produce a lesion.
c Damage to the cervical, thoracic and cauda equina areas of the cord have all been reported.

There is no evidence that any form of airway management is more or less likely to be associated with spinal cord damage than the other.

Patients with cervical disease, whether it may be essentially due to stenosis of the spinal canal (disc protrusions, spondylosis, ossification of the posterior longitudinal ligament, rheumatoid, tumours, haematomas) or instability (rheumatoid, trauma, tumours) should be regarded as at risk of spinal cord injury during general anaesthesia. Awake intubation and positioning may be sometimes the best way of trying to ensure that the position in which the patient is placed for surgery is optimal. However, it must be recognized that this is not a guarantee that injury will not occur. Monitoring of spinal evoked motor and sensory potentials is re-assuring for anaesthetists and surgeons, but has not been shown to *prevent* injury.

Key points

- Difficult laryngoscopy is common if the craniocervical junction is involved.
- Post-operative airway obstruction is not uncommon.

- If the patient says he '*can't breathe*' – re-intubation is usually required.
- S_aO_2 and stridor are not reliable signs.
- Spinal cord injury during anaesthesia does occur, the causation is sometimes uncertain, but airway management is an unlikely cause.

Further reading

Blumenthal S, Nadig M, Gerber C, Borgeat A. Severe airway obstruction during arthroscopic shoulder surgery. *Anesthesiology* 2003; **99**: 1455–1456.

Calder I, Calder J, Crockard HA. Difficult direct laryngoscopy in patients with cervical spine disease. *Anaesthesia* 1995; **50**: 756–763.

Calder I, Picard J, Chapman M, O'Sullevan C, Crockard HA. Mouth opening – a new angle. *Anesthesiology* 2003; **99**: 799–801.

Crosby E. Airway management after upper cervical spine injury: what have we learned? *Can J Anaesth* 2002; **49**: 733–744.

Donaldson III WF, Heil BV, Donaldson VP *et al.* The effect of airway maneuvers on the unstable C1–C2 segment. A cadaver study. *Spine* 1997; **22**: 1215–1218.

McCleod ADM, Calder I. Spinal cord injury and direct laryngoscopy – the legend lives on. *Br J Anaesth* 2000; **84**: 705–709.

Sagi HC, Beutler W. Airway complications associated with surgery on the anterior cervical spine. *Spine* 2002; **9**: 949–953.

Weglinski MR, Berge KH, Davis DH. New-onset neurologic deficits after general anesthesia for MRI. *Mayo Clin Proc* 2002; **77**: 101–103.

R. Vanner

Effects of aspiration

Aspiration is the process by which material is carried from the pharynx to the lower respiratory tract. The clinical outcome depends on the volume and nature of the aspirate, its distribution and the host defence mechanisms. The consequences can vary from relatively benign to fulminant acute respiratory failure and death. Aspiration of solids or semi-solids may cause airway obstruction. Aspiration of acidic gastric contents can cause a pneumonitis with bronchospasm and pulmonary oedema (Mendelson's Syndrome). A ventilation–perfusion mismatch will occur. In some patients worsening hypoxaemia may develop and lead to the adult respiratory distress syndrome (ARDS). Of those patients that aspirate 64% have no respiratory sequelae, 20% require ventilation on an intensive therapy unit (ITU) for more than 6 h and 5% die. If no symptoms or signs are present 2 h after an episode of aspiration, respiratory sequelae are unlikely.

Curtis Lester Mendelson 1913–2002

Mendelson was a gynaecologist in New York, until he abandoned the rat-race and became a general practitioner in the Bahamas at the age of 46. He continued to work there till the age of 77, when he retired to Florida. He made two nearly successful attempts to swim the English Channel and once caught and landed a 498-pound Marlin while fishing from a 10-ft skiff.

Diagnosis of aspiration

Symptoms: Most patients are unconscious and asymptomatic, but conscious patients will complain of breathing difficulty.

Signs: Dyspnoea and tachypnoea develop, often with a cough productive of pink frothy sputum. Tachycardia and hypotension are observed. The principal sign of aspiration is hypoxaemia. Even a few millilitres of saline instilled into the trachea will cause a temporary drop in oxygen saturation. Localized or diffuse wheeze and crackles may be heard on auscultation of the chest.

Investigations: Diffuse alveolar infiltrates usually in the lower lobes are apparent on the chest radiograph.

The risk of pulmonary aspiration

Aspiration occurs in 1 in 4000 anaesthetics for elective surgery and 1 in 900 for emergency surgery. If a tracheal tube is used then aspiration is just as likely after extubation as during induction.

It is generally agreed that patients presenting for elective surgery that have fasted of food for 6 h and clear drinks for 2 h (and do not fall into the high risk groups below) are at low risk of aspiration and that no particular precautions need to be taken to prevent the pulmonary aspiration of gastric contents. This is probably because the risk of morbidity from the precautions themselves outweighs the risks of aspiration in this group of patients.

Those patients with a higher risk of aspiration during anaesthesia are: those who are not fasted when they present for surgery; patients with delayed gastric emptying (bowel obstruction, upper gastrointestinal (GI) cancer, critical illness, acidosis, pain, opiates and cases of diabetes mellitus with an autonomic neuropathy or a high blood glucose); those patients with an incompetent lower oesophageal sphincter (patients with oesophagitis, previous oesophageal surgery or women more than 20 weeks pregnant). It is these higher risk patients that need precautions to prevent regurgitation and aspiration pneumonitis.

Although oesophagitis is often symptomatic, occasionally it is not. Patients with a small hiatus hernia often have no oesophagitis, have a normal lower oesophageal sphincter pressure and are not in a high-risk group unless they have symptoms of regurgitation. Light anaesthesia during airway manipulation causing coughing and straining can predispose to regurgitation and patients with a difficult airway have a higher incidence of aspiration.

Precautions

The anaesthetic techniques described are mainly directed at preventing regurgitation of refluxed gastric contents from the oesophagus into the pharynx during the induction of anaesthesia, as well as the use of a tracheal tube (cuffed in adults) to prevent aspiration if regurgitation occurs after induction. In children uncuffed tubes are used and in those at risk a nasogastric tube is necessary to empty the stomach. In patients with bowel obstruction, where gastric contents can be 1 l or more, a nasogastric tube should be inserted and aspirated before induction if not already passed. In other patients likely to have a full stomach, an orogastric tube can be passed during anaesthesia to empty the stomach before extubation as aspiration can occur in the early post-operative period. Extubation should always be performed when the patient is awake and lying on their side, not in the supine position. The larynx is not able to protect the lungs from aspiration for a period of time following extubation and the patient should remain on their side until fully awake and talking. Although the lateral position should allow pharyngeal contents to empty out before they are aspirated into the trachea, suction apparatus should always be at hand to assist this process during the recovery period. In pregnant patients at term additional precautions are taken to

reduce the acidity of gastric contents, as otherwise they have a mean pH of 1.4.

Anaesthetic technique

In 1956 the Association of Anaesthetists had collected 1000 reports of anaesthetic deaths and 110 of them were from pulmonary aspiration of stomach contents. This frequently occurred during induction of general anaesthesia, especially when muscle relaxant drugs were used. Anaesthetic techniques were developed to prevent aspiration in those patients at risk and they included; emptying the stomach beforehand, intravenous (i.v.) induction with the head up tilt position and also inhalational induction in the lateral and head down position (see below).

In 1961 Sellick described cricoid pressure as a technique used to prevent regurgitation of stomach contents during the induction of general anaesthesia. Despite no randomized controlled trials demonstrating the benefit or otherwise it was brought into widespread practice in the UK by 1970 and largely replaced the other techniques. Since then, cricoid pressure has become a routine part of anaesthetic practice for those patients at risk of aspiration in combination with pre-oxygenation, an i.v. induction, fast onset muscle relaxation and tracheal intubation. This technique has been termed rapid sequence induction. A recent survey of all the maternity units in the UK has shown that all of them routinely apply cricoid pressure during induction of general anaesthesia.

The term 'rapid sequence' relates to the technique of reducing the time between loss of consciousness, onset of neuromuscular blockade and placement of the tracheal tube. This reduces the chance of retching with cricoid pressure. Generous doses of i.v. anaesthetic suppress reflexes such as retching and hypertension but can also reduce the blood pressure in some patients. The normal signs of loss of consciousness should be sought before the onset of neuromuscular blockade in order to reduce the incidence of awareness. To improve cardiovascular stability a large dose of opiates can allow the reduction in dose of the i.v. anaesthetic but depresses respiration (see below).

Complications of cricoid pressure

Too much force applied to the awake patient has caused retching and deaths from both aspiration and ruptured oesophagus.

Difficulties with intubation can be caused by cricoid pressure: if the force is applied to the thyroid cartilage, if the larynx is pushed laterally to the left or if too much force is used, which compresses the airway. When cricoid pressure is applied properly with a force of up to 30 N (3 kg) the view at laryngoscopy is improved, even though the larynx can be distorted, compared to when no cricoid pressure is used. However, if only the epiglottis can be seen then the slight lateral displacement of the larynx, which is almost inevitable (up to 8 mm), will make the passage of a gum elastic bougie more difficult as this is normally passed in the midline.

Cricoid pressure can obstruct the airway and prevent ventilation of the lungs with a facemask and Guedel airway. This is proportional to the force applied as 30 N caused complete airway obstruction in 2% of patients whereas 40 N caused obstruction in 35%.

Do these risks outweigh the benefits?

There is no evidence of benefit for cricoid pressure as there have been no randomized controlled trials. There is some evidence that cricoid pressure reduces lower oesophageal sphincter pressure, which results in a reduction of oesophageal barrier pressure. Indeed, there are anecdotal reports in the literature of regurgitation occurring during induction of anaesthesia despite cricoid pressure. Three of twenty anaesthetic nurses or operating department practitioners questioned at our hospital have seen this once each during their careers. However, few things in medicine are 100% effective and there is circumstantial evidence that the incidence of aspiration has been dramatically reduced since the introduction of cricoid pressure in the late 1960s.

The confidential enquiries into maternal deaths in England and Wales in the 6 years 1958–1963 found 33 maternal deaths from aspiration. The trachea was intubated as a planned procedure in only five of these women. Following the recommendation published in 1963 that a tracheal tube should be used to protect the lungs, deaths from aspiration actually rose. In the years 1964–1969, 52 women died from aspiration, though in all but one intubation had been planned. The majority regurgitated on induction following thiopentone, suxamethonium and mask ventilation but before the trachea was intubated. None of them received cricoid pressure. Since cricoid pressure has been applied routinely deaths from aspiration have been few and usually confined to the early post-operative period. In 1945 Mendelson reported 66 cases of aspiration during general anaesthesia out of 44,016 pregnancies, two of whom died, while in 1996 Soreide reported four cases of aspiration during general anaesthesia out of 36,800 pregnancies, none of whom died. None of Mendelson's patients were intubated but in Soreide's series they were intubated and had cricoid pressure applied. Statistical analysis cannot be applied, as the number of general anaesthetics in each series was not reported. The increase of regional anaesthesia techniques and the routine use of antacid therapy may also account for reduced aspiration and mortality. A randomized controlled trial designed to answer the question of whether cricoid pressure reduces the frequency of aspiration would need to have large numbers due to the rarity of aspiration and might not be deemed ethical.

I suggest that we continue to use cricoid pressure, but apply it correctly and release it appropriately if airway problems occur, rather than abandon it and use other techniques, which also have no evidence of benefit, which might return us to the high incidence of death from aspiration in the 1960s. Aspiration despite cricoid pressure should not be seen as negligent practice. Whereas, aspiration without cricoid pressure in a high-risk case, might well be seen as negligent practice.

Failed intubation

If the airway is predicted or known to be difficult, awake fibre-optic intubation or spinal anaesthesia should be considered instead of a rapid sequence induction. Most failed intubations during a rapid sequence induction are therefore unexpected. It is important not to continue to try and intubate as oedema of the larynx may develop which could prevent ventilation. Three good attempts should be the limit which should include alternative laryngo-scope blades and a bougie. When only the epiglottis is seen, temporary release of cricoid pressure will allow the larynx to return to the midline and increase the chance of a bougie passed in the midline to enter the trachea. However, this is controversial as regurgitation may occur.

A failed intubation plan with the aim of maintaining oxygenation and awakening the patient should be initiated immediately. Waking the patient is the primary goal as suxamethonium usually starts to wear off in 3 min and cricoid pressure cannot be physically maintained for more than a few minutes because of fatigue.

Reduce the force of cricoid pressure by half in order to extend the time that cricoid pressure can be applied and to allow ventilation. Ventilate the lungs with a bag, mask and Guedel oral airway until the patient starts breathing. Once breathing commences, turn the patient onto their left side, tip the trolley head down, and release cricoid pressure. Spinal anaesthesia or awake fibre-optic intubation can then be considered. If surgery must proceed due to an urgent life threatening situation then either a facemask with a Guedel oral airway or the laryngeal mask airway (LMA) may be used to maintain the airway. The use of the ProSeal LMA has been recently described in this situation with positive pressure ventilation without a leak and passage of a gastric tube facilitated.

Can't intubate, can't ventilate

When the lungs cannot be ventilated cricoid pressure should be released completely to allow ventilation. If regurgitation occurs it is necessary to quickly perform oro-pharyngeal suction before attempting ventilation. If ventilation is still not possible the further airways that will then be necessary, such as the LMA, Combitube or the cricothyrotomy cannula, are all better placed without cricoid pressure applied.

Succinylcholine

Succinylcholine gives a rapid onset of muscle relaxation for intubation of the trachea and is used in most rapid sequence inductions. Although it can cause a rise in gastric pressure of up to 25 mmHg, lower oesophageal sphincter pressure increases by a similar amount probably due to the fasciculation of the crus of the diaphragm. Rocuronium also has a rapid onset and is argued by some to be superior, since the anaesthetist is under less time–pressure to complete intubation before the drug wears off. Furthermore, if intubation is difficult it allows better conditions for intubation, bag and mask ventilation, LMA insertion or cricothyrotomy as necessary without the complication of laryngospasm. This is controversial. Traditional teaching is not to even give another dose of succinylcholine if there are difficulties with intubation, the idea of using a long acting muscle relaxant does not therefore follow traditional teaching. If intubation fails, waking the patient up to await more senior assistance or to perform a different technique such as awake fibre-optic intubation or spinal anaesthesia is not possible. We have all heard of patients who have been in the 'can't intubate, can't ventilate' scenario that have started breathing, which has saved the day. However, these cases are difficult to find in the literature. Also, cricoid pressure can only be physically maintained for a few minutes due to fatigue.

If the airway is known to be easy rocuronium is a reasonable alternative to succinylcholine. For a similar reason, opioid drugs are not usually given during a rapid sequence induction unless the airway is known to be easy. In late pregnancy, as plasma cholinesterase concentration is low, succinylcholine can have a prolonged effect in those that are heterozygote for atypical cholinesterase. This can occur in about 5% of the population.

Correct technique for cricoid pressure

The anaesthetic assistant should practise the correct forces on weighing scales beforehand. The anaesthetist should be confident that the anaesthetic assistant knows the anatomical landmarks of the cricoid cartilage. Although Sellick suggested that the patient's head and neck should be extended, it should rest on a pillow as intubation is easier and cricoid pressure has since been shown to be just as effective in this position. Sellick also suggested that any nasogastric tube should be removed, but it has been shown that cricoid pressure is more effective when the nasogastric tube is left in place. It should be aspirated and then left open to atmospheric pressure by connecting to a bag to allow venting of gas or liquid to reduce any increase in gastric pressure during induction.

Firstly, the anaesthetic machine must be checked including suction apparatus, laryngoscopes and the tipping trolley or bed. Full monitoring of the patient is next including attachment of the capnograph to the anaesthetic circuit. Following i.v. access pre-oxygenation for 3 min may commence. This should be with an oxygen flow of at least $8\,l\,min^{-1}$ if a re-breathing circuit such as the Bain circuit or a circle system are used. The bag must distend with each breath and the mask must have a seal on the face.

Before i.v. induction, lightly applied cricoid pressure should be started with a force of 10 N (1 kg), after loss of consciousness the force is increased to 30 N (3 kg). Forces of 20 N or more are not tolerated when awake and may cause patients to retch and vomit. Normally the assistant applies cricoid pressure with their dominant hand as this can be maintained more accurately and for longer (3–5 min). There is no evidence that a bimanual technique, with the assistant's other hand supporting the patient's neck, improves the view at laryngoscopy when the correct forces are applied. The assistant's other hand is best kept free to assist with a difficult intubation if necessary. The only place for a bimanual technique is with a suspected fracture of the cervical spine when the counter pressure reduces movement of the spine together with manual in-line stabilization.

Alternatives to cricoid pressure

Cricoid pressure is contra-indicated in some situations. Occasionally patients with a barrel-shaped chest with chronic obstructive pulmonary disease have their cricoid cartilage positioned behind their sternum and cricoid pressure cannot be applied. It is said that patients with trauma to the neck and a fractured larynx and cricoid ring is a contra-indication. Large foreign bodies stuck at the level of the cricopharyngeus may prevent the occlusion of the hypopharynx with cricoid pressure. Children will not tolerate cricoid pressure awake and it must be applied after the onset of anaesthesia.

A gaseous induction in the left lateral position with the trolley in a slight head down position with intubation during deep anaesthesia has been described. The upper oesophageal sphincter does not relax with this technique as it does with i.v. thiopentone or muscle relaxant drugs. If regurgitation does occur it can come out of the mouth or be suctioned and will not necessarily be aspirated uphill into the trachea. This technique is useful with the post-operative bleeding tonsil, especially in children, where time can be taken to identify structures during laryngoscopy, which may not be obvious due to blood and oedema. Only anaesthetists experienced in intubation in the lateral position should use this technique, as over-extension of the neck is easily done which can make laryngoscopy difficult. The anaesthetist should kneel at the left corner of the trolley not at the top in order to avoid this problem. The technique should therefore be practised regularly in elective patients. Intubation in the right lateral position is difficult.

Induction in the steeply head up position has been described and was used in the 1960s, the anaesthetist had to stand on a chair. The theory was that the pharynx would be 20 cm above the stomach and gastric pressure would be less than $20\,cmH_2O$. However, regurgitation and aspiration did sometimes occur as well as hypotension.

Awake fibre-optic intubation can be performed in someone with a full stomach who is thought to have a difficult airway. However, care must be taken not to topically anaesthetize the trachea in order to retain the cough reflex in case regurgitation and aspiration occur, which has been described. Spinal anaesthesia could also be considered if the airway is difficult, but is risky in cases such as a strangulated hernia with bowel obstruction as massive regurgitation with aspiration has occurred in the supine position despite the patient being awake.

'Classic' rapid sequence induction

- *Pre-oxygenation*   Once the set-up is ready, the patient is pre-oxygenated with a tight-fitting facemask, with a high flow of 100% oxygen. The reservoir bag should be distended and moved with respiration – if it is not distended the facemask has not made a seal around the mouth. Gas flows should be high enough ($10\,l\,min^{-1}$) to prevent re-breathing, which is a problem with both the Bain circuit and circle absorber systems. Preoxygenation should be for either 3–5 min of tidal volume breathing, 4–8 slow maximal vital capacity breaths or until the end-tidal oxygen is 90–91%. Towards the end of the pre-oxygenation period, the assistant should locate the cricoid cartilage with the fingers ready for cricoid pressure application. Apply 10 N force while the patient is awake.
- *Induction, paralysis and cricoid force*   A pre-determined dose of induction agent (classically thiopentone $5\,mg\,kg^{-1}$) is administered into a fast-flowing i.v. infusion followed by succinylcholine $1.5\,mg\,kg^{-1}$. Cricoid pressure is increased at the anaesthetist's request when the patient loses consciousness. The correct force is 30 N (the force required to register 3 kg on a weighing machine) and is applied by the assistant on the cricoid cartilage with the fingers of one hand, applying force to push the cricoid ring posteriorly. The cricoid ring is not squeezed between the fingers. The facemask position is maintained, without attempts at facemask ventilation, until the onset of paralysis which corresponds to the *end* of visible fasciculations. The patient is intubated by direct laryngoscopy. A long blade may be needed and a bougie is particularly helpful – it should be used early. Intubation attempts must be limited and further doses of succinylcholine should not be given.
- *Confirmation of correct tube position*   Correct placement of the tube in the trachea should be confirmed by the methods outlined in Chapter 9. Cricoid force is released when tracheal intubation has been confirmed and anaesthesia now continues as normal, with administration of non-depolarizing muscle relaxants when succinylcholine is wearing off. Do not use unnecessarily large tubes – 7.0 mm inner diameter (ID) is satisfactory.

Management of a case of suspected aspiration

If aspiration occurs, immediate pharyngeal suction of regurgitated material must be performed. The patient should be positioned on their side to prevent further aspiration. If the patient is unconscious, intubation and tracheal suction may be appropriate. Aspiration of food particles can cause airway obstruction at the level of the larynx, trachea or bronchi and laryngoscopy or bronchoscopy may be required for removal of solid material. Bronchial lavage is not helpful and may disseminate the aspirated material. If the patient is awake however, coughing is effective at expelling small fragments of particulate material. Bronchodilators may sometimes be helpful, but corticosteroids are of no proven benefit and may predispose to infection. Antibiotic treatment is usually not started unless an ineffective process is identified. Cardiovascular support may be needed initially with the sudden extravasation of fluid into the lung. Mechanical ventilation may be needed with worsening hypoxaemia in which case further lung injury from hyperoxia and barotrauma must be minimized. Mortality may be as high as 50% if ARDS develops.

Key points

- Pulmonary aspiration of gastric contents still causes anaesthetic related mortality.
- Aspiration occasionally occurs despite cricoid pressure and has been described with all the anaesthetic techniques used to try and protect the patient from aspiration.
- Rapid sequence induction of anaesthesia with cricoid pressure is usually the technique of choice for those at risk of aspiration.
- If a difficult intubation is anticipated, awake fibre-optic intubation or spinal anaesthesia should be considered instead.
- Cricoid pressure should be released in the can't intubate can't ventilate situation.
- Extubate patients at risk when they are awake in the lateral position.

Further reading

Awan R, Nolan JP, Cook TM. Use of a ProSeal laryngeal mask airway for airway maintenance during emergency Caesarean section after failed tracheal intubation. *Br J Anaesth* 2004; **92**: 144–145.

Brimacombe JR, Berry AM, White A. An algorithm for the use of the laryngeal mask airway during failed intubation in the patient with a full stomach. *Anesth Analg* 1993; **77**: 398–399.

Garrard A, Campbell AE, Turley A, Hall JE. The effect of mechanically-induced cricoid force on lower oesophageal sphincter pressure in anaesthetized patients. *Anaesthesia* 2004; **59**: 435–439.

Maltby JR. *Notable Names in Anaesthesia*. London: RSM Press, 2002.

Mendelson CL. The aspiration of stomach contents into the lungs during obstetric anesthesia. *Am J Obstet Gynecol* 1946; **52**: 191–205.

Soreide E, Bjornestad E, Steen PA. An audit of perioperative aspiration pneumonitis in gynaecological and obstetric patients. *Acta Anaesth Scand* 1996; **40**: 14–19.

Vanner RG, Asai T. Safe use of cricoid pressure. *Anaesthesia* 1999; **54**: 1–3.

Warner MA, Warner ME, Weber JG. Clinical significance of pulmonary aspiration during the perioperative period. *Anesthesiology* 1993; **78**: 56–62.

THE LOST AIRWAY 21

C. Frerk

Introduction

A trained anaesthetist rarely has significant difficulty in maintaining a patent airway and ventilating the patient's lungs. When difficulty occurs the degree of difficulty encountered covers a spectrum, at the far end of which is the situation where the patient is consuming oxygen faster than the anaesthetist can deliver it; for the purpose of this chapter this is the definition of the lost airway. Other terms are 'can't ventilate, can't intubate' (CVCI) or 'can't intubate, can't oxygenate' (CICO). This extreme situation is rare in elective general surgery with an incidence of $1:10,000$ to $1:50,000$. Diagnosis and management must be complete within minutes of the onset of the problem to have a chance of a successful outcome.

Pathophysiology

An adult patient requires $200-250\,\mathrm{ml\,min^{-1}}$ of oxygen to sustain life. After induction of anaesthesia if this amount of oxygen cannot be delivered to the patient's lungs they will use up their reserves over $1-2\,\mathrm{min}$ (longer if well preoxygenated, sooner in the obese or those with increased requirements) and then they will start to desaturate. Without intervention to increase oxygen delivery to the lungs the patient will die. How long an individual patient will survive will depend on many factors. Anecdotal accounts of death due to airway obstruction (judicial execution by hanging) suggest that about $10\,\mathrm{min}$ of complete airway obstruction will result in cardiac arrest.

Most general anaesthetic agents decrease upper airway tone tending to lead to compromise of the natural upper airway and minor degrees of difficulty with facemask ventilation around the time of induction of anaesthesia. The loss of tone associated with the use of neuromuscular blocking drugs is considerably greater than that seen with intravenous or volatile anaesthetic agents, potentially leading to greater compromise of the natural airway (especially where there is pre-existing difficulty). Another cause of difficulty with ventilation around the time of induction of anaesthesia is obstruction at the level of the larynx caused by laryngeal spasm. In this situation ventilation is likely to be improved by deepening anaesthesia or the administration of neuromuscular blocking drugs. Arguments have been made for and against neuromuscular blocking drugs in difficult ventilation. Traditional teaching remains that when difficulty with tracheal intubation or ventilation of the lungs is anticipated, muscle relaxants should not be given until the airway is secured.

Level of obstruction

If difficulty with facemask ventilation occurs around the time of induction of anaesthesia it is usually assumed that the level of the problem is with the patient's natural upper airway or difficulty with facemask application to the face. Some factors are known to be associated with difficulty with ventilation (obstructive sleep apnoea, obesity, facial hair, tumour, previous difficulty), but difficulty cannot always be predicted prior to induction of anaesthesia. Preoperative assessment has typically been targeted at tests to predict difficult laryngoscopy rather than difficulty with ventilation of the lungs and there are well known shortcomings with these assessment systems. American Society of Anesthesiologists (ASA) closed claims reviews show that a significant proportion of failed ventilation cases occur in patients where some difficulty has been predicted but for whom the anaesthetic plan has not taken account of the potential risks. In two thirds of reviewed cases, repeated non-surgical attempts at tracheal intubation were deemed responsible for the loss of the airway. Where difficulty is anticipated with either tracheal intubation or ventilation of the lungs a safe anaesthetic technique should be chosen which may involve avoiding general anaesthesia altogether, using a local or regional technique or performing awake intubation prior to general anaesthesia. Problems at other levels of the airway can give rise to failed ventilation.

Obstruction at larynx/pharynx

- *Loss of natural upper airway tone.*
- *External compression of natural airway (e.g. cricoid pressure)*
  The cricoid cartilage is the only complete cartilaginous ring encircling the trachea and it has been assumed that correctly applied pressure (30 N) to the cricoid cartilage will occlude the oesophagus while leaving the trachea patent. However, the cricoid cartilage is much more deformable *in vivo* than was previously believed and forces of 30 N can narrow the airway and greater forces may occlude it, particularly in female patients. In a failed ventilation situation where cricoid pressure is being applied, the pressure should be reduced/removed to determine if this is the cause of the obstruction.
- *Airway device misplacement or occlusion*
  Laryngeal mask airways, tracheal tubes and other airway devices can be misplaced or function incorrectly leading to failure to ventilate the lungs. One notable problem is with the tracheal cuff which when inflated may occlude the lumen of the tube or herniate over the distal end. Rarely these devices can become occluded in the manufacturing process or during cleaning and resterilizing, resulting in a lost airway even though the device is placed correctly.

Proximal to the larynx

- *Breathing system malfunction, misassembly or occlusion*
  There are many reports of stuck valves, faulty scavenging systems and incorrectly assembled breathing systems leading to the inability to ventilate the lungs. Breathing systems, filters, angle pieces and catheter mounts can also become occluded with similar consequences and luer lock caps, plastic from packaging, syringe plungers, rogue pieces of anaesthetic equipment and unidentified gelatinous materials have all been implicated in various reports of serious morbidity or death. Equipment faults leading to inability to ventilate the lungs are entirely avoidable by performing a thorough preoperative equipment check. Although rare as a cause of failed ventilation, serious hypoxic injury and death have occurred as a result of equipment faults that could have been identified preoperatively. The Association of Anaesthetists of Great Britain and Ireland (AAGBI) guidelines (*Checking Anaesthetic Equipment*, 3: 2004) recommend that the whole breathing system including a new single-use filter, catheter mount and airway device are checked for patency immediately before use on *each* new patient.

Distal to the larynx

- *Severe bronchospasm/anaphylaxis*
  Anaphylaxis is both unpredictable and unavoidable. The incidence varies between 1:5000 for muscle relaxants and <1:10,000 for intravenous induction agents; 25% of such cases are associated with severe bronchospasm presenting as failure to ventilate the lungs with rapidly progressive hypoxia. Due to the timing and other associated symptoms, anaphylaxis is usually not difficult to diagnose. Treatment follows established guidelines from the AAGBI.
- *Mucus plugs.*
- *Tension pneumothorax.*

These distal problems, when severe, will give rise to failed ventilation. Antecedent history may direct the anaesthetist to one of these as the cause of the problem. Specific treatment will be determined by the suspected pathology.

Diagnosis

Loss of the airway is quite apparent once the saturations begin to fall but identifying loss of the airway before this happens gives longer for a definitive diagnosis to be made and for the correct course of action to be determined and put into place. Early recognition of the problem depends on identifying the pattern of decreased or absent chest movement and an absent or abnormal capnograph trace associated with unusual airway pressures. These signs are not specific for the cause of the problem but this may be apparent from the timing and/or nature of the difficulty. Airway pressures will be high when the airway is obstructed (subjective when ventilating by hand, monitored when using mechanical ventilators), but may be normal or low if the cause of airway loss is a misplaced tracheal tube; in this latter case airway pressures may still be unusual in that the expiratory pattern will often be atypical.

Making (or more accurately, accepting) the diagnosis is a difficult mental process. As discussed above, anaesthetists are used to some difficulty with airway maintenance and are skilled in a variety of techniques to improve the situation (jaw thrust, four handed ventilation, the use of airways, laryngeal masks and tracheal intubation). The only thing that distinguishes the lost airway from all these other cases is that the anaesthetist's usual armamentarium of techniques do not restore ventilation. A common feature in deaths due to the lost airway is that time is lost in denial – the situation is so rare that most anaesthetists will not have come across it before and the diagnosis is only accepted when the patient has become severely hypoxic and often when an agonal rhythm appears on the electrocardiograph (ECG). Training in the decision-making process to identify the lost airway early is needed, simulator based training is safe and has been shown to be effective for this purpose.

Management

Having made the diagnosis of a lost airway the first stage is to determine the site of difficulty while trying to ventilate the lungs with 100% oxygen. Knowledge of the patient's history, and of the drugs, techniques and equipment used in the period leading up to loss of the airway may lead the anaesthetist to an intuitive diagnosis of the cause of the problem. This allows definitive treatment which should resolve the problem. If an intuitive diagnosis is not possible, or if the management instituted is not successful, then a systematic approach needs to be adopted swiftly (Table 21.1):

- Breathing system blockage is reported to occur in 1 : 5 million anaesthetics. AAGBI guidelines

Table 21.1 Outline of causes and management of failed ventilation

Problem	Possible cause	Consider
Failed face mask	Breathing system failure Non-patent upper airway Laryngeal spasm	Self-inflating bag Oral airway, laryngeal mask Deepen anaesthesia
Failed face mask and laryngeal mask	Breathing system failure Non-patent upper airway Laryngeal spasm	Self-inflating bag Tracheal intubation Deepen anaesthesia
Failed ventilation via tracheal tube	Breathing system failure Blocked tracheal tube Tube in oesophagus Tracheal occlusion Severe bronchospasm Tension pneumothorax	Self-inflating bag Deflate cuff or remove tube Remove and reinsert Rare Intravenous adrenaline, salbutamol Needle decompression

(*Checking Anaesthetic Equipment*, 3: 2004) recommend having a self-inflating bag immediately available for just such an eventuality. An equipment problem can be rapidly excluded by connecting this bag directly to the anaesthetic face mask, tracheal tube or laryngeal mask airway (*excluding* all filters, catheter mounts and angle pieces).

- If a tracheal tube or laryngeal mask (or other airway conduit) has been placed this should be considered suspect, removed and ventilation confirmed with a face mask. If this is successful then the artificial airway conduit can be replaced with a new one and anaesthesia continued.

- If difficulty persists with a tracheal tube that has been seen to pass through the vocal cords and is not resolved by reverting to a face mask or laryngeal mask then the most likely cause for loss of the airway is a distal airway problem which should be treated accordingly. Knowing the antecedent history will determine the most appropriate course of action; recent chest trauma may suggest chest drains (needle decompression in the first instance), timing in relation to drugs administered along with other signs may suggest anaphylaxis requiring adrenaline. Rarely, unrecognized tracheal or anterior mediastinal pathology may be a cause of failed ventilation.

- In a patient where loss of the airway is unexpected and associated with total inability to apply facemask ventilation, ventilate via the laryngeal mask, visualize the vocal cords or to pass a tracheal tube the most likely diagnosis is of loss of the patient's natural upper airway leading to obstruction at that site. The treatment in this situation (after excluding cricoid pressure as the cause of difficulty) is emergency cricothyroidotomy.

Emergency cricothyroidotomy

The cricothyroid membrane (CTM) is the common site of emergency access to the trachea for oxygenation. It has several desirable features (Table 21.2). There are three types of cricothyroidotomy – small needle/cannula, large purpose-built cannula and

Table 21.2 Desirable features of the CTM

- Superficial, easily palpable
- Present in most patients
- Rarely calcifies
- Relatively avascular
- 1 cm *below* the vocal cords
- Usually large enough to take a 6.0 mm tube
- Cricoid ring holds the airway open
- Posterior lamina prevents inadvertent posterior wall puncture

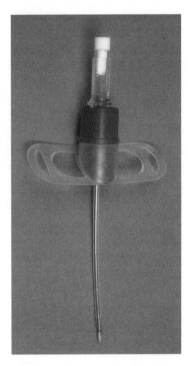

Figure 21.1 Ravussin style device for needle cricothyrotomy.

surgical. In general, cricothyroidotomy is quicker than tracheostomy.

Small needle

A 14G cannula or rigid needle (Figure 21.1) with an approximate internal diameter of 2 mm is placed through the CTM (Figure 21.2(a–e)) and directed caudally into the trachea (Table 21.3). Gas is aspirated freely from the cannula to confirm correct placement within the trachea. The small diameter

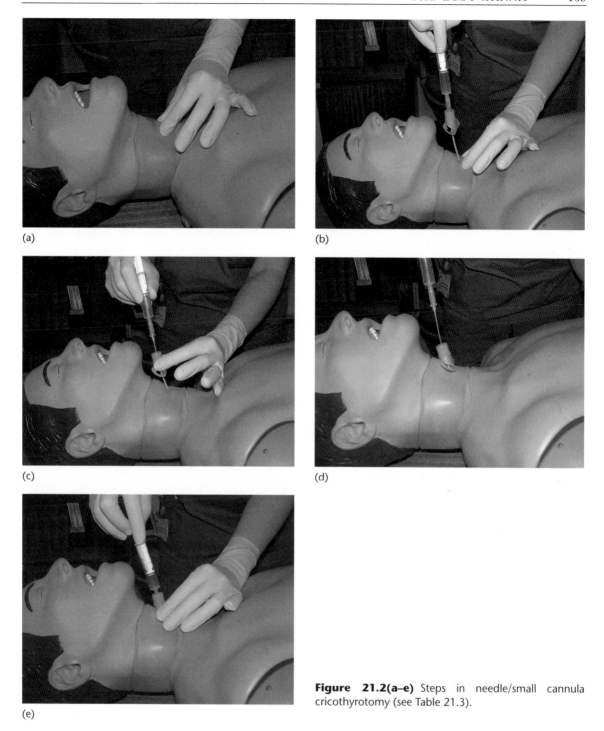

Figure 21.2(a–e) Steps in needle/small cannula cricothyrotomy (see Table 21.3).

limits gas flows such that exhalation of 500 ml takes over 30 s and adequate inspiratory gas flows require high-pressure oxygen. Using the anaesthetic breathing system with adjustable pressure limiting (APL) valve pressure of 70 cmH$_2$O results in a flow of about 80 ml s^{-1}, bypassing the breathing system valve and using the pressure of the back-bar relief valve (33 kPa) results in a flow of approximately 200 ml s^{-1} and pressures of 2–4 bar are required to provide inspiratory flows >500 ml s^{-1}. Since the normal

Table 21.3 Steps in emergency needle cricothyroidotomy

- Extend the chin and neck to improve access
- Place syringe on needle/cannula
- Identify CTM and stabilize larynx with one hand
- Insert needle through the CTM, aspirating to confirm intratracheal location
- Once in the trachea keep needle still
- Slide cannula off inserted needle
- Remove needle only when cannula fully inserted
- Aspirate free air through cannula to confirm correct placement
- Secure the cannula with hand initially or ties around neck later
- Apply short burst of high-pressure oxygen
- Watch chest rise appropriately *and* fall
- Maintain upper airway patency with laryngeal mask or oral airway for exhalation

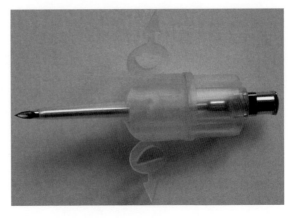

Figure 21.3 Quicktrach, large cannula-over-needle.

breathing system is not attached, capnography is not immediately available to confirm continued correct placement. Suctioning is not possible through the small cannula. Exhalation occurs through the upper airway which must be held open by a laryngeal mask or insertion of an oral airway with jaw thrust. Complications include incorrect placement in the pretracheal region or in the oesophagus, bleeding, damage to surrounding vascular structures and barotrauma.

Large purpose-built cannula

If the cannula has an internal diameter >4 mm, passive exhalation of 500 ml takes about 6 s and adequate inspiratory gas flows can be achieved with the pressures generated within a standard anaesthetic breathing system. Exhalation can occur through the cannula, suctioning is possible through it and capnography can be used to confirm placement within the trachea. The Quicktrach (Figure 21.3) is a rigid cannula–over–needle with a diameter of 4 mm, the Melker system is a Seldinger technique inserting a 6 mm cuffed or uncuffed tube. The Portex MiniTrach kit inserts a 4 mm tube which can be connected to either a 15 mm connector or a luer lock for high-pressure oxygenation. Complications include bleeding, damage to the surrounding structures and misplacement of the cannula outside the trachea leading to failure of the technique.

Surgical

In the basic technique, a horizontal incision is made through the CTM with a scalpel and a 6.0 mm tube placed into the trachea. The scalpel handle can be used to quickly dilate the incision to make certain that the airway has been entered. Surgical mini-sets containing a blade, blunt forceps for track dilation and a cricoid hook to hold the anterior wall of the trachea during tube insertion are available. The technique may be rapid and effective, allowing a cuffed tube to be inserted.

Choosing which technique

One type of cricothyroidotomy kit should be chosen for a hospital and be made available in all areas (operating theatres, the accident and emergency department and the obstetric unit). Training in the use of that particular device on a mannikin is essential to gain familiarity with the device and to maintain skills after initial training. A cadaver trial of the time to first ventilation taken by inexperienced intensive therapy unit (ITU) physicians, comparing surgical cricothyrotomy and a Seldinger technique found that *the two methods had equally poor performance*. Tracheal access was achieved only in 70% of the surgical group and 60% of the Seldinger group. A variety of algorithms have been published in the USA and Canada, and many UK hospitals have developed local protocols. The Difficult Airway Society has recently developed national guidelines for the UK and the 2004 guidelines for failed ventilation are shown in Figure 21.4.

Failed intubation and difficult ventilation (other than laryngospasm)

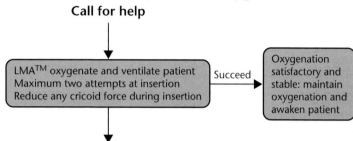

1. Face mask
2. Oxygenate and ventilate patient
3. Maximum head extension
4. Maximum jaw thrust
5. Assistance with mask seal
6. Oral ±6 mm nasal airway
7. Reduce cricoid force – if necessary

Failed oxygenation with face mask (e.g. $SpO_2 < 90\%$ with F_iO_2 1.0)

Call for help

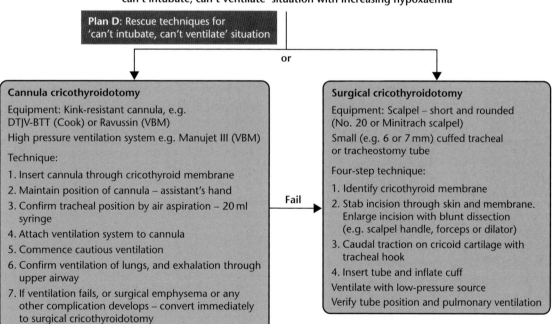

LMA™ oxygenate and ventilate patient
Maximum two attempts at insertion
Reduce any cricoid force during insertion

Succeed →

Oxygenation satisfactory and stable: maintain oxygenation and awaken patient

'can't intubate, can't ventilate' situation with increasing hypoxaemia

Plan D: Rescue techniques for 'can't intubate, can't ventilate' situation

or

Cannula cricothyroidotomy

Equipment: Kink-resistant cannula, e.g. DTJV-BTT (Cook) or Ravussin (VBM)

High pressure ventilation system e.g. Manujet III (VBM)

Technique:

1. Insert cannula through cricothyroid membrane
2. Maintain position of cannula – assistant's hand
3. Confirm tracheal position by air aspiration – 20 ml syringe
4. Attach ventilation system to cannula
5. Commence cautious ventilation
6. Confirm ventilation of lungs, and exhalation through upper airway
7. If ventilation fails, or surgical emphysema or any other complication develops – convert immediately to surgical cricothyroidotomy

Fail →

Surgical cricothyroidotomy

Equipment: Scalpel – short and rounded (No. 20 or Minitrach scalpel)

Small (e.g. 6 or 7 mm) cuffed tracheal or tracheostomy tube

Four-step technique:

1. Identify cricothyroid membrane
2. Stab incision through skin and membrane. Enlarge incision with blunt dissection (e.g. scalpel handle, forceps or dilator)
3. Caudal traction on cricoid cartilage with tracheal hook
4. Insert tube and inflate cuff

Ventilate with low-pressure source

Verify tube position and pulmonary ventilation

Notes:
1. These techniques can have serious complications – use only in life-threatening situations
2. Convert to definitive airway as soon as possible
3. Postoperative management – see other difficult airway guidelines and flow-charts
4. Four millimetres cannula with low-pressure ventilation may be successful in patient breathing spontaneously

Difficult Airway Society Guidelines Flow-chart 2004 (use with DAS guidelines paper)

Figure 21.4 Difficult Airway Society UK algorithm for management of failed intubation, increasing hypoxaemia and difficult ventilation (other than laryngospasm) in the paralysed anaesthetized patient, the 'can't intubate, can't ventilate' situation (www.das.uk.com). LMA: laryngeal mask airway.

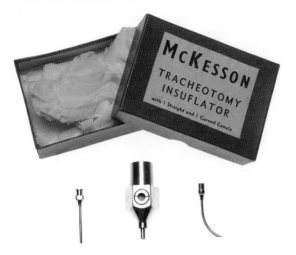

Figure 21.5 McKesson emergency airway access needles with 15 mm connector.

Table 21.4 Complications (occurring in up to 20% of cases in some series) associated with emergency cricothyroidotomy

- Bleeding – immediate or delayed
- Barotrauma with high-pressure oxygen
  - Surgical emphysema
  - Pneumothorax
- Device misplacement
  - Anterior to trachea
  - Lateral to trachea
  - through posterior wall
- Laryngeal trauma
- Tracheal stenosis
- Death

It is known from research published in the 1950s that insufflation of oxygen through a needle cricothyroidotomy can reverse falling oxygen saturations. A variety of devices were developed on the strength of this work (Figure 21.5) and this relatively simple technique has been the fall-back plan of many anaesthetists since then. The needle can be placed expectantly and anaesthetists are used to inserting cannulae, but high-pressure oxygen is required giving rise to the possibility of barotrauma, exhalation must be possible through the upper airway and there is the problem of ensuring that the cannula remains in the trachea. In a number of reported cases anaesthetists have proceeded to surgical cricothyroidotomy despite having already inserted a cricothyroid cannula because of doubts over the placement of that cannula. It is important that the cricothyroid kit contains appropriate needles, preferably those designed for the purpose, syringe for insertion and some mechanism for providing high-pressure oxygen with coherent connectors throughout. It is inappropriate to consider a self-assembly kit from items usually found in the anaesthetic room.

While *elective* transtracheal jet ventilation via small cannulae is well established, some consider the emergency use of this technique to be too hazardous. A short wide bore cannula through which to-and-fro ventilation can occur with a low-pressure breathing system may be the device of choice although some have queried whether an uncuffed 4–5 mm tube can effectively resuscitate an adult if the upper airway is patent. Seldinger techniques are slower than percutaneous cannula-over-needle techniques, but the insertion of a cuffed tube would appear to be most desirable. With the increased popularity of percutaneous tracheostomy many anaesthetists are gaining the transferable skills needed to minimize the risks associated with emergency access to the trachea (Table 21.4).

Key points

- The lost airway is an emergency, time is limited.
- A thorough machine/equipment check (including all components of the breathing system and airway devices) should be performed prior to each anaesthetic.
- Making the diagnosis is a difficult mental process and time is often lost in denial.
- Equipment problems and distal airway problems should be rapidly excluded.
- Emergency cricothyroidotomy can be a difficult practical procedure, the sooner it is started, the more likely is re-establishment of the airway before irreversible hypoxic injury occurs.
- As it is rare the necessary mental and practical skills cannot be learnt on routine operating lists. Mannikin/simulator training is required.

Further reading

Bell D. Avoiding adverse outcomes when faced with 'difficulty with ventilation'. *Anaesthesia* 2003; **58**: 945–948.

Benumof JL, Scheller MS. The importance of transtracheal jet ventilation in the management of the difficult airway. *Anesthesiology* 1989; **71**: 769–778.

Caplan RA, Posner KL, Ward RJ, Cheney FW. Adverse respiratory events in anesthesia: a closed claims analysis. *Anesthesiology* 1990; **72**: 828–833.

Carter JA. Checking anaesthetic equipment and the Expert Group on Blocked Anaesthetic Tubing (EGBAT). *Anaesthesia* 2004; **59**: 105–107.

Crosby ET, Cooper RM, Douglas MJ *et al*. The unanticipated difficult airway with recommendations for management. *Can J Anaesth* 1998; **45**: 757–776.

Eisenburger P, Laezika K, List M, Wilfing A *et al*. Comparison of conventional surgical versus Seldinger techniques of emergency cricothyrotomy performed by inexperienced clinicians. *Anesthesiology* 2000; **92**: 687–690.

Miller CG. Management of the difficult intubation in closed malpractice claims. *Am Soc Anesthesiol Newslett* 2000; **64**: 1–6.

Rosenblatt WH, Wagner PJ, Ovassapian A, Kain ZN. Practice patterns in managing the difficult airway by anesthesiologists in the United States. *Anesth Analg* 1998; **87**: 153–157.

Vanner R. Emergency cricothyroidotomy. *Curr Anaesth Crit Care* 2001; **12**: 238–243.

I. Calder

Anaesthetic trauma

Dental damage

Dental damage most often occurs during direct laryngoscopy, the upper incisors are most frequently damaged and diseased or restored teeth are most at risk. Avulsed teeth should be stored in milk or saline (never water) for possible re-implantation by dental surgeons. Dental damage is the most common cause of a civil action against anaesthetists, and a careful assessment of pre-anaesthetic dental condition may prevent subsequent claims.

Naso/pharyngeal/oesophageal damage

Damage to the nasal turbinates, even complete avulsion, or perforation of the nasopharyngeal mucosa can occur during nasal intubation. Intubation over a guide, such as a suction catheter or endoscope is recommended. Sepsis following pharyngeal or oesophageal perforation during intubation is one of the principal causes of anaesthetic mortality. Urgent treatment is required (antibiotics and drainage) and patients in whom perforation is suspected should be closely observed for symptoms (sore throat, cervical or chest pain, dysphagia) and signs (fever).

Glottic damage

A persistent sore throat, weak cough and dysphonia should prompt a laryngoscopy. Possible causes include subluxation of an arytenoid cartilage (Figure 22.2), vocal cord palsy or haematoma (Figure 22.3). The diagnosis of arytenoid subluxation has followed intubations that were regarded as easy by the anaesthetist, but Paulsen *et al.* failed to induce arytenoid

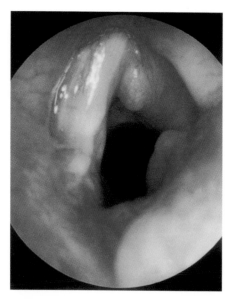

Figure 22.1 Avulsion of vocal cord by tracheal tube. This injury occurred during neonatal resuscitation. (Reprinted, with permission from Benjamin B. *Endolaryngeal Surgery*. Taylor and Francis Books Ltd (Martin Dunitz), London 1998).

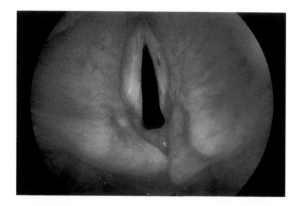

Figure 22.2 Right arytenoid cartilage subluxation. The right vocal cord was immobile. (Reprinted, with permission from Benjamin B. *Endolaryngeal Surgery*. Taylor and Francis Books Ltd (Martin Dunitz), London 1998).

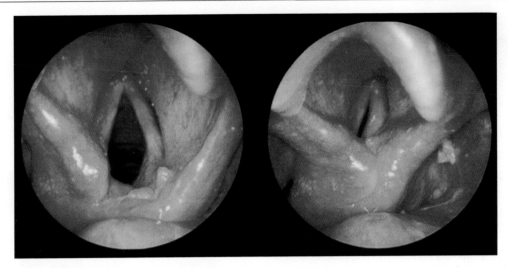

Figure 22.3 Left vocal cord palsy. (Reprinted, with permission from Benjamin B. *Endolaryngeal Surgery*. Taylor and Francis Books Ltd (Martin Dunitz), London 1998).

subluxation in cadaver specimens despite strenuous efforts. They proposed that trauma at intubation causes 'cricoarytenoid joint dysfunction'.

Tracheal damage

Acute

Perforation or rupture can occur during intubation and is not always obvious immediately. The cardinal sign is subcutaneous air. A tracheal tube may need to be placed below a rupture. The use of fibreoptic placement of two microlaryngoscopy tubes has been reported.

Chronic

Prolonged intubation will cause damage. The duration required depends on the type and particularly the size of tube, cuff design and inflation pressure and the presence of aggravating factors such as infection, poor tissue perfusion, acid reflux, and excessive movement during suction and coughing. The sites commonly affected are the medial aspects of the cricoarytenoid joints, the posterior glottis and the subglottic trachea. The injuries seen are oedema, granulation tissue formation (Figure 22.4)

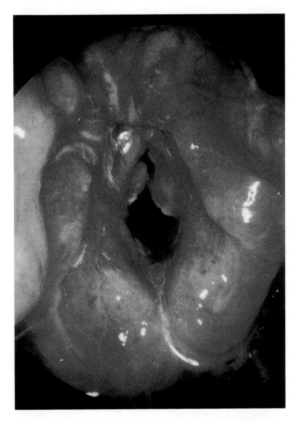

Figure 22.4 Oedema and granulation tissue formation due to prolonged intubation and reflux of gastric acid. (Reprinted, with permission from Benjamin B. *Endolaryngeal Surgery*. Taylor and Francis Books Ltd (Martin Dunitz), London 1998).

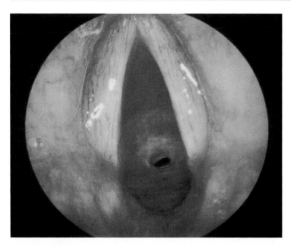

Figure 22.5 Tracheal stenosis following prolonged intubation. (Reprinted, with permission from Benjamin B. *Endolaryngeal Surgery*. Taylor and Francis Books Ltd (Martin Dunitz), London 1998).

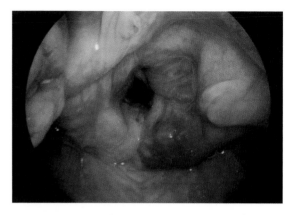

Figure 22.6 Laryngeal damage due to being hit in the throat with a baseball bat. (Reprinted with permission from Benjamin B. *Endolaryngeal Surgery*. Taylor and Francis Books Ltd (Martin Dunitz), London 1998).

and ulceration in the acute stage, followed by stenosis (Figure 22.5).

The period for which intubation should be allowed has not been established. In general, tracheostomy is preferred if more than a week of intubation will be required. In children much longer periods can be tolerated.

Non-anaesthetic trauma

Blunt trauma

Facio-maxillary injuries can cause airway obstruction. The most likely are bilateral mandibular fractures and Le Fort III maxillary fractures where there is cranio-facial separation. Bleeding from these fractures can be severe, and aspiration of blood and tissue, bone and tooth fragments can occur.

Laryngotracheal injuries are uncommon, with an estimated incidence of only one per 1000 trauma victims (Figure 22.6). Diagnosis is often difficult and delayed. Symptoms vary from obvious airway obstruction to virtually none. Patients with severe airway trauma often succumb before reaching hospital. The thyroid cartilage is more often damaged than the cricoid, but damage to the cricoid is more often associated with airway obstruction. The

principal sign of airway damage is subcutaneous air, and fibreoptic laryngoscopy is the most important examination. Computerized tomography (CT) scan can be helpful.

Indications for surgical exploration

- Airway obstruction.
- Uncontrolled air leak.
- Exposed cartilage.
- Immobile cord.
- Associated soft tissue injury to the neck.

Tracheostomy is often the safest way to control the airway, but some patients can be managed with a tracheal tube. A team approach with ear, nose and throat (ENT) surgeons is required.

Penetrating trauma

A retrospective study found that 40% of patients with penetrating neck trauma eventually required tracheal intubation. As with other penetrating wounds, the severity of injury depends largely on the velocity of the penetrating object, so that stab wounds have a better outlook than missile injuries. Penetrating neck wounds are usually described according to the 'zone' of entry.

Patients with extensive airway injury may have few external signs. Subcutaneous air is again the cardinal

Zone	Frequency %	Limits	Airway implications
1	5	Clavicle to cricoid cartilage	Often require intubation because of great vessel injury
2	80	Cricoid to angle of mandible	Mostly require intubation for surgical exploration; approximately one-third need emergency airway intervention
3	15	Angle of mandible to base of skull	Less likely to need airway intervention

sign. Radiographs or CT scan may reveal injury. Approximately 25% of penetrating wounds also have oesophageal trauma, which may present late.

Thermal trauma

There are three sites of airway injury:

a *Oropharyngeal burn*: Swelling can cause airway obstruction. This is likely if there are full thickness facial and anterior cervical burns. Maximal swelling occurs 12 h after the burn.

b *Glottic burn*: Any sign of airway obstruction should prompt immediate intubation. Carbon in the nares, mouth or pharynx makes a glottic burn likely. Fibreoptic or indirect laryngoscopy should be performed and if there is any sign of glottic involvement, it is best to insert a tracheal tube as sudden obstruction can occur.

c *Smoke inhalation*: This accounts for 50% of fire-related deaths. Altered consciousness, hypoxaemia and expiratory wheeze are the principal signs.

Key points

- Dental damage is the most frequent cause of a civil action against anaesthetists.
- Perforation of the pharynx/oesophagus/trachea may not be apparent at the time and is an important cause of mortality.
- Subcutaneous air is the principal sign of airway perforation.
- Patients with suspected airway injury must be closely observed as airway obstruction can be rapid.

Further reading

Chadwick RG, Lindsay SM. Dental injuries during general anaesthesia. *Br Dent J* 1996; **180**: 255–258.

Cicala RS. The traumatized airway. In: Benumof JL (Ed.). *Airway Management – Principles and Practice*. St Louis: Mosby, 1996; pp. 736–759.

Domino KB, Posner KL, Caplan RA, Cheney FW. Airway injury during anesthesia: a closed claims analysis. *Anesthesiology* 1999; **91**: 1703–1711.

Kannan S, Chestnut N, McBride G. Intubating LMA guided awake fibreoptic intubation in severe maxillofacial injury. *Can J Anaesth* 2000; **47**: 989–991.

Kuttenberger JJ, Hardt N, Schlegel C. Diagnosis and initial management of laryngotracheal injuries associated with facial fractures. *J Craniomaxillofac Surg* 2004; **32**: 80–84.

Paulsen FP, Rudert HH, Tillmann BN. New insights into the pathomechanism of post intubation arytenoid subluxation. *Anesthesiology* 1999; **91**: 659–666.

Shearer VE, Giesecke AH. Airway management for patients with penetrating neck trauma: a retrospective study. *Anesth Analg* 1993; **77**: 1135–1138.

Stannard K, Wells J, Cokis C. Tracheal rupture following endotracheal intubation. *Anaesth Intens Care* 2003; **31**: 588–591.

Stout DM, Bishop MJ, Dwersteg JF, Cullen BF. Correlation of endotracheal tube size with sore throat and hoarseness following general anaesthesia. *Anesthesiology* 1987; **67**: 419–421.

I. Calder

Mortality due to anaesthesia

The UK is probably comparable to other developed countries where the mortality has been found to be approximately 1:10,000. UK anaesthetists will administer approximately 18,000–30,000 anaesthetics in their careers, so the chances of being involved in a tragedy are not negligible.

Causes of anaesthetic mortality

Mistakes or complications associated with drug administration cause the majority of deaths (approximately 40%). Deaths due to airway management have declined and in the last reported study from the USA, problems with airway management caused the same number of fatalities as central venous line insertion (20%).

Causes of airway mortality

The causes continue to be loss of airway during attempts at intubation, perforation of the pharynx, oesophagus or trachea, and oesophageal intubation. Rarer causes are aspiration of stomach contents, laryngospasm and bronchospasm.

Loss of airway at intubation

The mechanism is unclear but the scenario is well recognized – a patient, who was initially possible to ventilate with a mask, becomes impossible to ventilate after repeated attempts to intubate. Possible causes are swelling of tissues due to trauma, laryngospasm, operator fatigue and panic. The message is clear – do not make repeated fruitless attempts to intubate. Aim to make one 'optimal best attempt' with all factors properly arranged.

Perforation of pharynx/oesophagus or trachea

The cause of death is usually sepsis following the development of mediastinitis or cervical abscess. The mortality rate from mediastinitis is about 20%. Acute airway obstruction or respiratory failure can result from surgical oedema or pneumothorax. Only half of the perforations are recognized (pneumothorax or subcutaneous air) at the time. Perforation can occur during easy intubation, but is strongly associated with difficult intubation. Patients who have been difficult to intubate (and their carers) should be warned to report symptoms of mediastinitis, as early treatment (drainage and antibiotics) is vital.

Mediastinitis: signs and symptoms	
Early	Sore throat, deep cervical or chest pain, cough
Later	Fever, dysphagia, dyspnoea

Oesophageal intubation

Deaths continue to occur. It is vital to continually consider the diagnosis and apply more than one method of confirmation of tracheal placement.

Medico-legal aspects

Physicians are increasingly exposed to legal actions. The use of suspension from duties and dismissal has increased. Civil actions and criminal accusations have all become more frequent. At least three anaesthetists have been convicted of manslaughter. The public and those charged with patient safety are more inclined to report practitioners to the General Medical Council. For an insight into the feelings of families who suspect they have been the victims of medical negligence, read 'Wrongful Death' by Sandra Gilbert.

Civil actions for negligence

The legal criteria for a finding of negligence are the following:

- The existence of a duty of care owed by one person to another.
- Breach of the duty of care.
- Foreseeable injury occurring as a consequence of the breach.

In private medical practice an action can also be brought for failure to comply with a 'contract', where an offer to treat has been accepted and a 'consideration' has been paid.

Criminal accusations

It is rare, but not unknown, for anaesthetists to use their skills to murder (where there is intention to kill or cause serious injury). The accusation of causing death by 'involuntary manslaughter' (where the defendant caused the death but without any intention to kill or cause serious injury) is becoming more common. The criteria for a finding of involuntary manslaughter are the following:

- The existence of a duty.
- Breach of the duty causing death.
- Gross negligence, which a jury considers, justifies a criminal conviction.

The criterion for 'gross negligence' is one of the following:

- The defendant was indifferent to an obvious risk of injury to health.
- Had actual foresight of the risk, but determined nonetheless to run it.

Bungling anaesthetist jailed for killing boy

AN anaesthetist who admitted killing a 14-year-old boy during a routine dental procedure was jailed for six months yesterday.

Dr Prabhakar Gadgil, 65, mixed up two tubes so patient Bradley Miller was given nitrous oxide or 'laughing gas' instead of oxygen.

As a result, the youngster, who suffered from the rare Goldenhar syndrome, which affects bone structure, suffocated during the procedure to remove a milk tooth.

Sentencing Gadgil at Sheffield Crown Court, Mr Justice Poole said: 'This offence was one of the most gross negligence. I have concluded, albeit with regret, that I would be failing in my public duty if I did not pass a custodial sentence.'

Gadgil, of Dewsbury, West Yorkshire, pleaded guilty to manslaughter. Bradley died at the Victoria House dental practice in Barnsley in 1997.

Earlier this month, dentist Neville Bainsbridge, 65, of Barnsley, who had also been charged with manslaughter, walked free after prosecutors decided the charge should be left on file.

Robert Smith QC, prosecuting, said:

'There is simply no excuse for such a fundamental mistake. It should have been detected if the dentist or Gadgil checked the equipment before it was used that day.'

He added that Bradley's medical condition meant he had a restricted airway which made resuscitation difficult.

'Neither the dentist nor Dr Gadgil asked about Bradley's medical history. The failure to take a history was a serious omission,' said Mr Smith.

'There were a whole series of errors and incidents of substandard management of safety procedures that led to this tragedy.'

Defending, John Goldring QC, said Gadgil was a 'decent, understanding and sensitive man' who was shattered by Bradley's death.

'He has taken all the responsibility for what happened but is quite clear that he is not solely to blame,' he said.

'He has not worked since the tragedy and will not work again. He will be struck off and is a broken man.'

Following Bradley's death, the General Dental Council issued new guidelines on the use of general anaesthesia to dentists throughout the country.

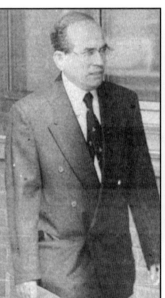
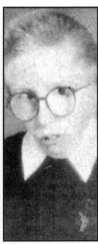

Dr. Prabhakar Gadgil (left) mixed up oxygen and nitrous oxide tubes while Bradley Miller (above) was in the dentist's chair

Reprinted with permission from The Metro newspaper (Associated Metro Ltd).

- The defendant appreciated the risk and intended to avoid it, but displayed such a high degree of negligence in the attempted avoidance as the jury considered justified conviction.
- The defendant displayed inattention or failure to advert a serious risk, which went beyond 'mere inadvertence' in respect of an obvious and important matter, which the defendant's duty demanded he should address.

The conviction rate is low, possibly because of difficulties in proving that the medical error caused the death. The level of proof must be 'beyond reasonable doubt' whereas 'on the balance of probabilities' is sufficient in a civil action. Anaesthetists have been convicted of manslaughter after a ventilator became disconnected when the anaesthetist was absent, and after a child with Goldenhar's syndrome was anaesthetized in a dental practice.

Standard of care

The standard required by medical practitioners is determined by judicial analysis of professional opinion.

Bolam test

The 'Bolam' test (named from the case in which the principle was first enunciated): a doctor will not be deemed negligent if he is acting in accordance with the opinion of a responsible body of medical practitioners, skilled and practised in that art. This test has been refined by stipulating that the medical opinion on which the court is invited to rely must also be 'reasonable'. This means that the court may find a doctor negligent even though he was following the procedures adopted by other doctors, if those procedures are unjustified by medical facts. The court must also apply the standard that pertained at the time of the events, not at the time of the trial.

Guidelines

Deviation from an accepted guideline or protocol *without good reason* is difficult to defend. However, the courts recognize that guidelines indicate an accepted course of practice, rather than a final arbiter of professional standards. It would otherwise be difficult to make advances in medical practice.

Key points

- Mortality due to airway management has fallen.
- Persistent attempts to intubate can result in loss of the airway.
- The possibility of perforation of the airway must be considered, especially after difficult intubation.
- Remember that your actions may be scrutinized by legal authorities.

Further reading

Arbous MS, Grobbee DE, van Kleef JW *et al*. Mortality associated with anaesthesia: a qualitative analysis to identify risk factors. *Anaesthesia* 2001; **56**: 1141–1153.

Biboulet P, Aubas P, Dubourdieu J *et al*. Fatal and non fatal cardiac arrests related to anesthesia. *Can J Anaesth* 2001; **48**: 326–332.

Branthwaite M, Beresford N. *Law for Doctors: Principles and Practice*, 2nd edition. The Royal Society of Medicine Press, 2003.

Caplan RA, Posner KL. Medical-legal considerations: the ASA closed claims project. In: Benumof JL (Ed.). *Airway Management, Principles and Practice*. St Louis: Mosby-Year Book Inc, 1996; pp. 944–955.

Domino KB, Posner KL, Caplan RA, Cheney FW. Airway injury during anesthesia: a closed claims analysis. *Anesthesiology* 1999; **91**: 1703–1711.

Fasting S, Gisvold SE. Serious intraoperative problems – a five year review of 83, 844 anesthetics. *Can J Anaesth* 2002; **49**: 545–553.

Gilbert S. *Wrongful Death: A Memoir*. New York/London: WW Norton & Co, 1997.

Jenkins K, Baker AB. Consent and anaesthetic risk. *Anaesthesia* 2003; **58**: 962–984.

Kawashima Y, Takahashi S, Suzuki M *et al*. Anesthesia-related mortality and morbidity over a 5-year period in 2,363,038 patients in Japan. *Acta Anaesthesiol Scand* 2003; **47**: 809–817.

Newland MC, Ellis SJ, Lydiatt CA *et al*. Anesthetic-related cardiac arrest and its mortality: a report covering 72,959 anesthetics over 10 years from a US teaching hospital. *Anesthesiology* 2002; **97**: 108–115.

Peters J. Recording electrocardiograms can be dangerous. *Anesthesiology* 2003; **99**: 1225–1227.

A. Patel & V. Mitchell

Difficult airway management problems are encountered more commonly during anaesthesia for ear, nose and throat (ENT) and maxillofacial procedures than probably any other branch of surgery. Surgery varies from high volume cases such as tonsillectomy and dento-alveolar surgery to complex head and neck cancer and craniofacial surgery. For a successful outcome these shared airway procedures require thorough pre-operative evaluation and close co-operation between anaesthetist and surgeon with an understanding of each other's problems and knowledge of specialist equipment.

General ENT and maxillofacial procedures

Airway management for ENT and maxillofacial procedures needs to take account of specific problems and a number of techniques may be useful (Table 24.1):

- Once surgery has commenced the anaesthetist is remote from the airway making adjustments to the airway more difficult and disruptive.
- Head and neck positioning for surgery and movements during surgery require a secure airway.
- For nasal and intraoral surgery the airway requires protection by soiling from blood and debris.

Table 24.1 Techniques available for general ENT and maxillofacial procedures

1   Face mask for simple ear procedures
2   Nasal mask for dental procedures
3   Oral tracheal intubation
4   Nasal tracheal intubation
5   LMA or FLMA

- Oropharyngeal and nasopharyngeal packs should be specifically recorded and accounted for at the end of the procedure.
- Direct inspection and suction clearance of blood and debris from the oro–nasopharynx should be undertaken at the end of the procedure.

Face mask

Until the introduction of the laryngeal mask airway (LMA) many simple ear procedures were undertaken with a face mask. The increased use of the LMA, compared to a face mask, for simple ear procedures is due to its ability to provide a clearer airway with a more effective airtight seal allowing better ventilation and monitoring of tidal gases. The anaesthetist's hands are also freed and factors which make facemask anaesthesia difficult, for example the edentulous bearded patient, have little impact on the quality of the airway with an LMA. Oxygen saturations are also higher, there is less pollution and surgical conditions have been shown to be superior for minor ear surgery in children as there is less movement of the surgical field.

Nasal mask

Nasal masks (Goldman or McKesson) are used to maintain anaesthesia for simple dental extractions particularly in children. Conventionally carried out in the dental chair, children are anaesthetized in the sitting position with either sevoflurane or halothane inhalation or by intravenous propofol. The anaesthetist stands behind the chair holding the nasal mask while supporting the patients jaw. The dentist inserts a mouth prop and a pack, which isolates the oropharynx preventing mouth breeding. The surgery is short and relatively straightforward. At the end of the procedure the patient is positioned on their side on a trolley for recovery.

Successful dental chair anaesthesia is dependent on a skilled anaesthetist and a skilled operator who can perform multiple extractions rapidly and has insight into the problems of the shared airway.

Oral tracheal tube

Tracheal tubes are commonly employed in ENT and maxillofacial procedures. Reinforced tubes are useful for procedures where head and neck movements or extreme positioning are anticipated for surgery. South facing oral tubes are particularly suitable for surgery involving the pharynx where a surgical gag is used.

Nasal tracheal tube

Nasal tracheal tubes are the mainstay of maxillofacial anaesthesia. They are easier to insert where a fibreoptic intubation is necessary, lend themselves to a blind insertion technique, are well tolerated once *in situ* and easily secured on the forehead so that surgical access is optimized. North facing nasal tubes are preferred as they can be fixed in place with strapping over the forehead without obscuring the bony contours of the face and pressure on the nostril can be avoided.

LMA/flexible LMA

Tracheal intubation has traditionally been the cornerstone of good anaesthetic practice in ENT surgery but more recently the advantages of the flexible LMA (FLMA) have been realized and its use in ENT and maxillofacial surgery increased. The successful use of the FLMA requires the acquisition of a wide range of new skills for the anaesthetist, surgeon and recovery room staff with a significant learning curve. The advantages of the FLMA over a tracheal tube are the avoidance of laryngoscopy for placement, less invasion of the respiratory tract, the avoidance of muscle relaxants and the risks of endobronchial or oesophageal intubation. The FLMA is tolerated at lighter levels of anaesthesia compared to a tracheal tube and the incidence of laryngeal spasm, sore throat, cardiovascular

responses to insertion and removal, and coughing, straining and breath holding during emergence are all significantly reduced.

This improved airway recovery profile is particularly important in these patients who have one of the highest incidences of airway recovery problems. A major advantage of the FLMA is that it can be left in place to secure the airway during the recovery period until return of the patient's protective reflexes. This avoids the dilemma faced by the anaesthetist using tracheal intubation of whether to extubate 'deep' and leave an unprotected airway, or extubate 'light' and have a patient more at risk of coughing, straining and breath holding. The improved recovery profile can also be utilized in patients who have undergone tracheal intubation by exchange of the tracheal tube for an LMA at the end of surgery, leaving the LMA as a conduit for recovery.

Airway management for laryngoscopy

Laryngoscopy is unique in that both anaesthetist and surgeon wish to work in the same anatomical field. The anaesthetist is concerned with adequate oxygenation, removal of carbon dioxide, maintenance of an adequate airway and the prevention of soiling of the tracheobronchial tree, while the surgeon requires an adequate view of a clear motionless operating field. For success, close co-operation and communication between anaesthetist and surgeon is essential with an anaesthetic and surgical plan discussed and agreed.

The ideal anaesthetic technique (Table 24.2) for all laryngoscopy procedures does not exist. The technique chosen will be dependent on the patient's general condition, the size, mobility and location of the lesion and surgical requirements including the use of a laser. The presence of a cuffed tracheal tube, while providing control of the airway and preventing aspiration, may obscure a glottic lesion (Figure 24.1) and is not laser safe. A cuffed laser tube provides some protection against laser-induced airway fires but has a greater external diameter to internal diameter

Table 24.2 The ideal anaesthetic technique for laryngoscopy

- Simple to use
- Provide complete control of the airway with no risk of aspiration
- Control ventilation with adequate oxygenation and carbon dioxide removal
- Provide smooth induction and maintenance of anaesthesia
- Provide a clear motionless surgical field, free of secretions
- Not impose time restrictions on the surgeon
- Not be associated with the risk of airway fire or cardiovascular instability
- Allow safe emergence with no coughing, bucking, breath holding or laryngospasm
- Produce a pain free, comfortable, alert patient with minimal hangover effects

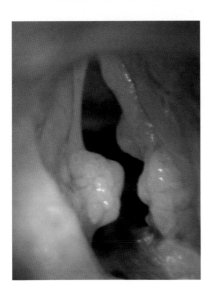

Figure 24.1 Papillomata on posterior third of both vocal cords: tracheal tube will impair surgical access.

Table 24.3 Vocal cord pathology

• Cysts	• Haemangiomas
• Polyps	• Renkies oedema
• Nodules	• Microweb
• Sulcus	• Post-operative scarring or stenosis
• Granulomas	• Congenital lesions
• Papillomas	• Malignant tumours

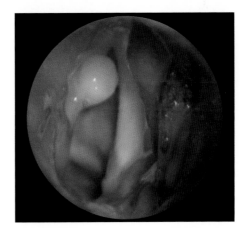

Figure 24.2 Polyp on anterior third of left vocal cord.

ratio and may obscure laryngeal lesions. Jet ventilation techniques require specialist equipment and knowledge, an understanding of their limitations and do not protect the airway from soiling.

Pre-operative assessment

Pre-operative assessment should aim to identify the probable vocal cord pathology, size, mobility, vascularity and location of the lesion. Patients presenting for laryngoscopy vary from young otherwise fit and well individuals, with voice changes secondary to benign vocal cord pathology (e.g. small nodules and polyps), to elderly, heavy smokers with chronic obstructive pulmonary disease presenting with voice changes, dysphagia and stridor caused by glottic carcinoma (Table 24.3, Figures 24.2 and 24.3).

A history of previous endoscopic procedures and outcome should be noted. Dysphagia, best breathing position, breathing pattern during sleep, voice changes and stridor give an indication of the severity of the disease. Patients may have no obvious stridor on initial examination but it may become apparent as the patient lies down, with changes from their best breathing position or on minimal exertion. Inspiratory stridor is usually associated with lesions above the glottis, whereas expiratory stridor is usually seen with lesions below the glottis. The severity and size of lesions at glottic level are assessed by

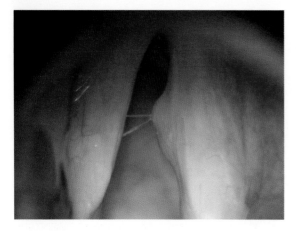

Figure 24.3 Nodule on middle third of right vocal cord.

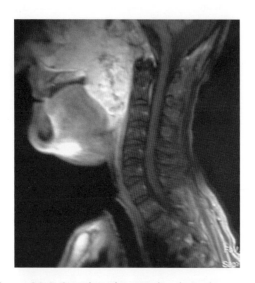

Figure 24.4 Complete pharyngeal occlusion by tumour: note end-tracheostome.

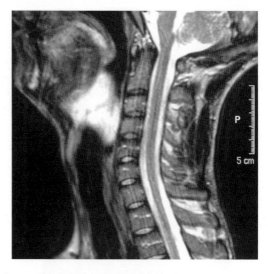

Figure 24.5 Tumour of tongue base.

direct or indirect laryngoscopy undertaken by surgeons in an outpatient setting; a photograph of the findings is often recorded in the notes and should be assessed. Surgical principles dictate that whenever a disease process impinges on the airway, its extent should be determined by computed tomography (CT), magnetic resonance imaging (MRI) or chest radiography whenever possible. Reviewing such scans with the surgeon is very rewarding, and is of particular value in assessment of subglottic or tracheal pathology (Figures 24.4–24.7).

An assessment of the size of the lesion gives an indication of potential airflow obstruction. Stridor indicates a significantly narrowed airway. In the adult, stridor implies an airway diameter of less than 4–5 mm, but the absence of stridor *does not* exclude a significantly narrowed airway. An assessment of the mobility of lesions (e.g. multiple large vocal cord polyps or papillomata) is important to identify those lesions that can potentially obstruct the airway following induction of anaesthesia due to the loss of supporting tone in the larynx. Mobile lesions if located in the supraglottis can obstruct the airway or make visualization of the laryngeal inlet difficult. Subglottic lesions (Figure 24.8) may allow a good view of the laryngeal inlet but cause difficulty during the passage of a tracheal tube or during jet ventilation.

Anaesthesia for laryngoscopy

For the majority of benign vocal cord lesions and early malignant lesions, airway obstruction is not a feature. Where airway obstruction is anticipated the anaesthetic plan will change (see below).

Anaesthetic techniques can be broadly classified into two groups. First 'closed' systems in which a cuffed tracheal tube is employed with protection of the lower airway and secondly, 'open' systems in which a cuffed tracheal tube is absent and employ either

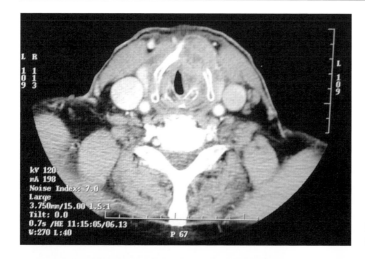

Figure 24.6 Glottic laryngeal cancer with destruction of left thyroid cartilage (Stage T4).

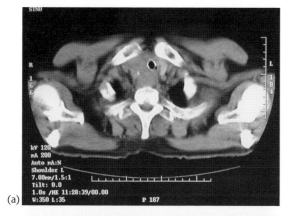

(a)

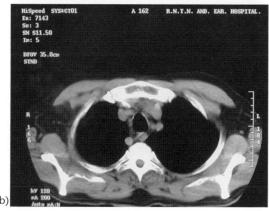

(b)

Figure 24.7 Subglottic stenosis with 3 mm airway (a) and normal distal trachea (b).

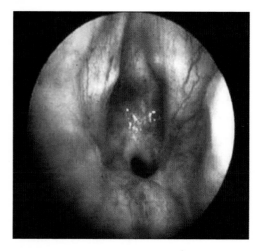

Figure 24.8 Subglottic stenosis.

spontaneous ventilation/insufflation techniques or muscle paralysis and jet ventilation.

The decision to use a 'closed' or 'open' technique will depend on the experience of the anaesthetist, the experience of the surgeon, the equipment available, the requirements for surgical access, the size, mobility and location of the lesion and its vascularity. The technique chosen for any given procedure is not absolute and may have to change as surgical and anaesthetic requirements change. For example, an open system utilizing jet ventilation on a lesion thought to be relatively avascular, may change to a closed system employing a cuffed tracheal tube if the lesion is bleeding significantly with the risk of soiling of the tracheobronchial tree. Conversely a system employing a cuffed tracheal tube may have to change during surgery to an open system if the tracheal tube overlies a lesion making surgery very difficult or impossible.

Table 24.4 Closed anaesthetic system

Advantages
1 Protection of the lower airway
2 Control of the airway
3 Control of ventilation
4 Minimal pollution by volatile agents
5 Routine technique for all anaesthetists

Disadvantages
1 Limitation of visibility and surgical access
2 Risk of laser airway fire
3 Risk of air entrapment and pneumothorax/ hypotension with small tubes
4 Risk of high inflation pressures and inadequate ventilation

Table 24.5 Open anaesthetic system

Advantages
1 Complete laryngeal visualization
2 Minimal risk of tube-related trauma to the glottis
3 Laser safety

Disadvantages
1 Unprotected lower airway
2 Require specialist equipment, knowledge and experience

Induction of anaesthesia

An intravenous induction technique is suitable for the vast majority of benign and early malignant glottic lesions in which airway obstruction is not anticipated. After pre-oxygenation and intravenous induction of anaesthesia, manual bag mask ventilation is confirmed before the administration of muscle relaxants appropriate to the length of surgery. Laryngoscopy is undertaken to visualize the larynx, establish laryngoscopy grade and administer topical anaesthesia (lignocaine). This helps cardiovascular stability, reduction of airway reflexes and smooth recovery. Confirmation of pathology is important because the disease may have progressed since the last outpatient visit and the anaesthetic plan may have to change. After induction of anaesthesia, during surgery, both closed and open systems are employed. Closed systems are familiar, using a cuffed microlaryngoscopy tube (ID 5 mm) or laser tube (see Chapter 7) and have advantages and disadvantages (Table 24.4).

Open systems

Open systems are common in head and neck surgery and will be described in more detail. They have advantages and disadvantages (Table 24.5) and include three main techniques:

- spontaneous ventilation/insufflation
- intermittent apnoea
- jet ventilation.

Spontaneous ventilation/insufflation technique

Spontaneous ventilation and insufflation techniques are useful in the removal of foreign bodies, evaluation of airway dynamics (tracheomalacia) and relatively fixed lesions (glottic, subglottic stenosis). Both techniques require a spontaneously breathing patient and allow a clear view of an unobstructed glottis.

Inhalational induction is commenced with sevoflurane or halothane in 100% oxygen. At a suitable depth of anaesthesia as assessed by clinical observations on the rate and depth of respiration, pupil size, eye reflexes, blood pressure and heart rate changes, laryngoscopy is undertaken and topical lignocaine is administered above, below and at the level of the vocal cords. 100% oxygen is administered by face mask with spontaneous ventilation and anaesthesia continued with inhalational (insufflation) or an intravenous anaesthetic technique (propofol). At a suitable depth of anaesthesia again assessed by clinical observations, the surgeon undertakes rigid laryngoscopy or bronchoscopy.

Insufflation of anaesthetic gases and agents can be via a number of routes:

- Small catheter introduced into the nasopharynx and placed above the laryngeal opening.
- Tracheal tube cut short and placed through the nasopharynx emerging just beyond the soft palate.
- Nasopharyngeal airway.
- Side arm or channel of a laryngoscope or bronchoscope.

Movements of the vocal cords are minimal or absent during a spontaneously breathing technique

Table 24.6 Limitations of spontaneously breathing/insufflation technique

- No control over ventilation
- Loss of protective airway reflexes and the potential for airway soiling
- Theatre pollution when volatile agents are used

Table 24.7 Intermittent apnoea technique

Advantages
1 Immobile, unobstructed surgical field
2 Inherent safety in the use of a laser with the potential fuel source (tracheal tube) removed

Disadvantages
1 Variable levels of anaesthesia
2 Interruption to surgery for reintubation
3 Potential trauma through multiple reintubation
4 The risk of aspiration of blood and debris with the tracheal tube removed

provided an adequate level of anaesthesia is maintained. If the depth of anaesthesia is too light, the vocal cords may move, the patient may cough or laryngospasm occur. If the depth of anaesthesia is too great the patient may become apnoeic with cardiovascular instability. Careful observations throughout the procedure, noting movements, respiratory rate and depth, cardiovascular stability and constant observation for unobstructed breathing are vital, with the concentration of volatile anaesthetic or intravenous anaesthetic adjusted accordingly. The technique has limitations (Table 24.6).

Intermittent apnoea

Intermittent apnoea techniques (Table 24.7) have been described for the laser resection of juvenile laryngeal papillomatosis, where the presence of a tracheal tube obstructs surgery. Following induction of general anaesthesia and confirmation of ventilation by face mask, muscle relaxants are administered followed by tracheal intubation. The patient is hyperventilated with a volatile anaesthetic agent in 100% oxygen. The tracheal tube is then removed, leaving the surgeon a clear, unobstructed, immobile surgical field. After an apnoeic period of typically 2–3 min, surgery is stopped, the tracheal

tube is reinserted and the patient hyperventilated once more.

Jet ventilation

Jet ventilation techniques involve the intermittent administration of high-pressure jets of air, oxygen or air–oxygen mixtures with entrainment of room air. Sanders in 1967 first described a jet ventilation technique using a 16-G jet placed down the side arm of a rigid bronchoscope relying on air entrainment to continue ventilation with an open bronchoscope. Sanders used intermittent jets of oxygen (rate 8 per minute, 3.5 bar driving pressure) to entrain air and showed the technique maintained supranormal oxygen partial pressure with no rise in the carbon dioxide pressure. Since 1967, modification to Sanders original jet ventilation technique have been made for endoscopic airway surgery. These modifications include the *site* at which the jet of gas emerges (supraglottic, subglottic, transtracheal – see Figure 24.9) and the *frequency* of jet ventilation (low frequency less than 1 Hz, high frequency more than 1 Hz).

High-frequency jet ventilation techniques typically use rates around 100–150 per minute. This allows:

- Continuous expiratory flow of air, enhancing the removal of fragments of blood and debris from the airway.
- Reduced peak and mean airway pressures (compared with low frequency) with improved cardiovascular stability.
- Enhanced diffusion and interregional mixing (compared with low frequency) within the lungs resulting in more efficient ventilation.

These advantages are of particular importance in patients with significant lung disease and obesity. High-frequency jet ventilators must have incorporated alarms and automatic interruption of jet flow when preset pause pressure limits have been reached (i.e. blockage of entrainment and exhalation have occurred).

The techniques are suitable for the vast majority of benign glottic pathology and early malignancy where airway obstruction is not anticipated. A typical jet ventilation technique will include preoxygenation followed by intravenous induction. At a suitable depth of anaesthesia manual confirmation of mask ventilation is made before administration of muscle relaxants. Laryngoscopy is undertaken and topical lignocaine administered. Facemask ventilation is continued with 100% oxygen and when the surgeon is ready a rigid (suspension) laryngoscope is sited onto which a jetting needle has been attached in preparation for supraglottic jet ventilation. Alternatively, an LMA can be inserted after induction and used to ventilate the patient with 100% oxygen until the surgeon is ready to site the laryngoscope. Maintenance of anaesthesia with a target-controlled infusion of propofol, supplemented by bolus administration or infusion of alfentanil or remifentanil is undertaken. At the end of surgery, the LMA is reinserted before antagonism of residual muscle relaxation and cessation of intravenous anaesthesia, to facilitate smooth emergence.

Supraglottic

Supraglottic jet ventilation (Table 24.8) describes a technique in which the jet of gas emerges in the supraglottis by attachment of a jetting needle to the rigid suspension laryngoscope. High- or low-frequency ventilation can be employed.

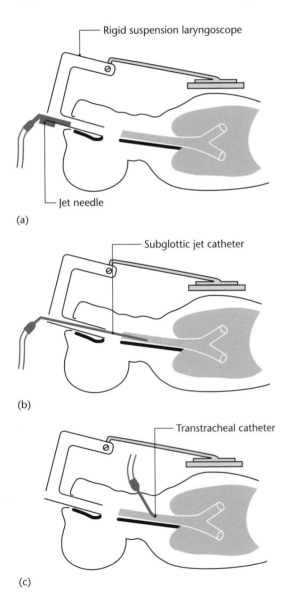

(a)

(b)

(c)

Figure 24.9 The three sites used for jet ventilation: (a) supraglottic jet ventilation, (b) subglottic jet ventilation and (c) transtracheal jet ventilation.

Table 24.8 Supraglottic jet ventilation

Advantages
1 Clear, unobstructed view for the surgeon
2 No risk of a laser-induced airway fire

Disadvantages
1 Risk of barotrauma with pneumomediastinum, pneumothorax and subcutaneous emphysema
2 Gastric distension with entrained air
3 Misalignment of the suspension laryngoscope or jetting needle resulting in poor ventilation
4 Blood and debris or fragments being blown into the distal trachea
5 Vibrations and movements of the vocal cords
6 Inability to monitor end tidal carbon dioxide concentration

---

Table 24.9 Subglottic jet ventilation

Advantages
1 Greater minute ventilation at any given driving pressure (compared to supraglottic)
2 Greater minute ventilation at any given frequency (compared to supraglottic)
3 Minimal influence on ventilation of laryngoscope alignment to the laryngotracheal axis
4 No vocal cord movements
5 No time constraints for the surgeon in the placement of the rigid laryngoscope

Disadvantages
1 Potential for a laser-induced airway fire (laser-resistant tubes are available, e.g. hunsaker)
2 Greater risk of barotrauma compared with supraglottic jet techniques

Subglottic

Subglottic jet ventilation (Table 24.9) involves the placement of a small (2–3 mm) catheter or specifically designed tube (Benjet, Hunsaker) through the glottis and into the trachea. This allows delivery of a jet of gas directly into the trachea.

Transtracheal

Elective transtracheal catheter placement under local anaesthesia in individuals with significant airway pathology or under general anaesthesia for elective laryngeal surgery has been described. Compared with supraglottic and subglottic jet techniques, transtracheal techniques carry the greatest risk of barotrauma and a high risk of subcutaneous emphysema. Its use for benign glottic pathology should be questioned with a careful evaluation of the potential risks and benefits made. Other potential problems include: blockage, kinking, infection, bleeding and failure to site the catheter.

Bronchoscopy

Bronchoscopy is indicated for examination of the tracheobronchial tree, biopsy and removal of bronchial lesions or foreign bodies. Bronchoscopy can be undertaken by either a flexible fibreoptic bronchoscope or a rigid bronchoscope. Rigid bronchoscopy allows better visualization, suctioning and control of bleeding. The principles of laryngoscopy apply equally to bronchoscopy, with good topical anaesthesia being essential. For inhaled foreign bodies generally a spontaneous/insufflation technique is employed to reduce the chances of further impaction into the tracheobronchial tree. For biopsy and removal of tracheobronchial lesions, ventilation can be either spontaneous or controlled. Controlled ventilation employs jet techniques as described by Sanders or high-frequency jet ventilation through the side arm of a rigid bronchoscope. As with all jet ventilation techniques careful observation of chest wall movements and listening to the sound produced during jet ventilation is essential. The sound changes during jet ventilation as the airway narrows or partial airway obstruction occurs.

Airway obstruction

Airway maintenance for patients presenting with airway obstruction is challenging and requires appropriate management by experienced anaesthetists and ENT surgeons. Three groups of patient can present with airway obstruction:

1 Infection (epiglottitis, supraglottitis, Ludwig's angina).
2 Glottic or subglottic stenosis following prolonged intubation.
3 Advanced upper airway tumours.

Infection

Epiglottitis

Acute epiglottitis (Figure 24.10) is an acute inflammatory disease of the epiglottis, arytenoids and aryepiglottic folds. The onset and progression of symptoms can be rapid leading to complete airway obstruction, hypoxaemia and death. It is usually seen in children aged between 2 and 6 years, although the condition can occur in infants, older children and adults. Epiglottitis is caused by a bacterial infection, typically haemophilus influenza type B, although the incidence of this is decreasing since the introduction of the Hib vaccine. Other causative organisms include beta-haemolytic streptococci, staphylococci, or pneumococci. In younger

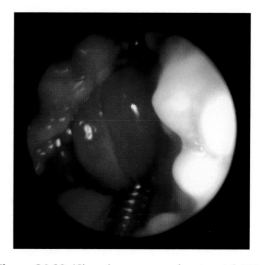

Figure 24.10 'Cherry' appearance of acute epiglottitis.

children it can be difficult to differentiate acute severe laryngotracheobronchitis (croup), which is a viral infection.

Classically the history is short with rapid deterioration. Adults and children present with a sore throat, fever, dysphagia, drooling, open mouth, muffled voice, respiratory distress, toxic and assume the tripod position with the child sitting and body leaning forward with the hands outstretched. The diagnosis is made on the history and examination of the child. Indirect laryngoscopy, oropharyngeal examination, intramuscular injections, placement of intravenous lines and lateral neck radiographs should not be undertaken without strong indication because further distress may precipitate complete airway obstruction.

The child should be moved to a quiet induction area with preparation for a difficult paediatric intubation and experienced anaesthetic and ENT surgeons summoned. Inhalational induction with sevoflurane or halothane in 100% oxygen is commenced with the child usually sitting or in the preferred position. Nitrous oxide is not used. Following inhalational induction, further monitoring and intravenous access are established as anaesthesia deepens. Intravenous fluids and atropine may be administered to reduce the likelihood of bradycardia with intubation. Laryngoscopy is undertaken at a suitable depth of anaesthesia and classically shows a swollen 'cherry-red' epiglottis with swelling of the aryepiglottic folds. With significant inflammation the glottic opening is not visible and the only clue may be expiratory gas bubbles during spontaneous ventilation or by gentle pressure on the child's chest. An uncuffed orotracheal tube usually 1–3 sizes smaller than predicted is placed with confirmation by auscultation and capnography. Once the child is stable this is replaced by a nasotracheal tube, which is less likely to become dislodged during the subsequent 24–48 h of ventilation on a paediatric intensive care unit. Throat and blood cultures are obtained, antibiotic therapy commenced and the child transferred to a paediatric intensive care unit. Usually within 24–48 h the child has become afebrile, appears well and a significant leak around the tracheal tube indicates that extubation is appropriate.

Ludwig's angina

This is a bilateral, rapidly spreading submandibular cellulitis, originating usually from the second or third molars and is due to streptococci or mixed oral floor. It was originally described by Wilhelm-Von-Ludwig in 1836 and angina implies the suffocating sensation. There is elevation and displacement of the tongue with firm, hard induration of the floor of the mouth and perioral oedema. The infection may spread posteriorly and cause trismus, occasionally involving deep cervical spaces and eventually the mediastinum. Patients present with pain, fever, trismus, dysphagia, difficulty swallowing and in severe cases maintaining an airway. Airway management involves the placement of a nasotracheal tube usually by means of an awake technique. Occasionally in severe disease a tracheostomy under local anaesthesia is indicated, although this carries the risk of mediastinitis. Surgery involves decompression of the fascial spaces and the removal of infected teeth. Patients remain intubated until upper airway oedema resolves.

Glottic/subglottic stenosis

In a very small proportion of patients following prolonged intubation, non-specific changes in the glottis and subglottis occur, including oedema and superficial ulceration resulting in granulation tissue, which progresses to firm scar tissue. The patients present with airway compromise many weeks or months after a period of intubation and may have been misdiagnosed as asthmatic. Surgical management of these patients involves:

- Laser resection of the stenotic region.
- Serial dilation of the glottic or subglottic stenosis.
- Insertion of soft stents to maintain airway patency and reduce the maturation of firm scar tissue.
- Topical chemotherapy (mitomycin) to reduce formation of scar tissue.
- For severe cases refractory to treatment, the stenotic sections are resected and 'end-to-end' tracheal anastomosis undertaken.

- For long sections of stenosis 'end-to-end' tracheal anastomosis will not be possible and tracheal homografts are grafted.

Airway management in these patients involves a spontaneous/insufflation technique or more commonly supraglottic jet ventilation technique.

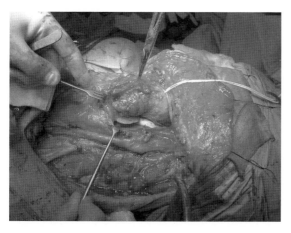

Figure 24.11 Tongue base tumour – operative view to show displacement of epiglottis.

Upper airway tumours

Upper airway tumours can be classified from the site at which they arise and extend.

Oropharyngeal

Oropharyngeal tumours can arise from any site within the oropharynx and include tumours arising from the tonsils, mandible, tongue, tongue base (Figure 24.11) and lateral oropharyngeal wall. With late presentation airway obstruction can be significant. Tumours arising from the vallecula, pyriform sinus or posterior cricoid oesophageal inlet regions are extra-laryngeal and are part of the oropharynx and hypopharynx.

Laryngeal

Laryngeal tumours are divided for the purposes of cancer treatment into supraglottic, glottic and subglottic, and are staged with a TNM (tumour, nodes and metastasis) classification (Table 24.10).

Table 24.10 The TNM staging of laryngeal cancer

Supraglottic

- T1: Tumour confined to site of origin with normal cord mobility
- T2: Tumour involving adjacent supraglottis
- T3: Tumour limited to larynx with fixation or extension or both to involve the post-cricoid area, medial wall of pyriform sinus, or pre-epiglottic space
- T4: Massive tumour extending beyond larynx to involve oropharynx, soft tissues of neck, or destruction of thyroid cartilage

Glottic

- T1: Confined to vocal cords with normal mobility (includes involvement of anterior or posterior commissure)
  - T1a: Unilateral involvement
  - T1b: Bilateral involvement
- T2: Supraglottic or subglottic extension of tumour or both with normal or impaired cord mobility
- T3: Tumour confined to larynx with cord fixation
- T4: Massive tumour with thyroid cartilage destruction or extension beyond confines of larynx or both
- N0: No regional lymph node metastasis
- N1: <3 cm, single ipsilateral lymph node
- N2: 3–6 cm
- M: Metastasis present

Subglottic

- T1: Tumour confined to the subglottic region
- T2: Tumour extension to vocal cords with normal or impaired cord mobility
- T3: Tumour confined to larynx with cord fixation
- T4: Massive tumour with cartilage destruction or extension beyond confines of larynx or both

Tracheal

The commonest primary malignant tumours of the trachea are squamous cell carcinomas and adeno cystic carcinomas. Secondary involvement of the trachea is usually by direct invasion from tumours of the thyroid gland, oesophagus, larynx and lung (Figure 24.12).

General principles in the pre-operative assessment of upper airway tumours

An assessment of the degree of airway obstruction can be made from a detailed history, examination and investigations. In the early stages of laryngeal tumours persistent hoarseness may be the only significant finding, while at the other extreme some patients can present late with large obstructing tumours, significant airway compromise and stridor at rest. The history should establish the severity of airway symptoms by the severity of dyspnoea, shortness of breath, hoarseness, haemoptysis,

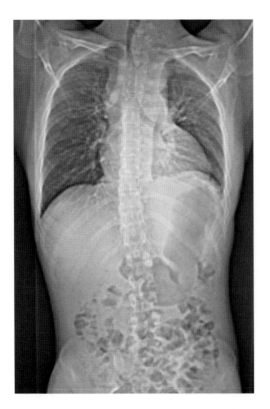

Figure 24.12 Mediastinal lymphadenopathy with upper tracheal narrowing.

dysphagia, secretions and drooling. The presence of stridor implies significant airway compromise, although its absence does not exclude significant airway compromise. Stridor may be absent in the patient at the bedside but may be significant on exertion, as the patient changes position or lies flat.

Over 80% of laryngeal and oropharyngeal tumours are found in men aged 40–65 years and over 97% of patients are smokers with a high alcohol intake. An assessment of cardiovascular and respiratory status should be made with reference to chronic obstructive pulmonary disease, bronchitis, hypertension and coronary artery disease. An alcohol withdrawal treatment should be established. Fibreoptic nasendoscopy undertaken by the ENT surgeons under local anaesthesia of the nose provides useful information on the extent of tumour extension over the airway. If a significant period of time has elapsed between the last flexible nasendoscopy, it should be repeated as the tumour may have extended further. Flexible nasendoscopy does not provide information on the distal extension of tumours. CT and MRI scans are required to build up a three-dimensional picture of the size, location and extension of the tumour.

Anaesthetic management for airway tumours

Anaesthetic management will be dependent on the site of the tumour, its size, its extension and degree of airway compromise but there are a number of standard approaches (Table 24.11).

Table 24.11 Management options with airway tumours

1   Intravenous induction of general anaesthesia
2   Inhalational induction with maintenance of spontaneous ventilation throughout
3   Inhalational induction of general anaesthesia with 'take over' of ventilation
4   Awake or asleep fibreoptic intubation
5   Transtracheal catheter placement under local anaesthesia and jet ventilation
6   Tracheostomy under local anaesthesia or general anaesthesia

Oropharyngeal tumours

Oropharyngeal tumours range from small early tonsillar carcinomas through to large obstructing tongue base tumours. For the majority of oral cavity tumours where there is no airway compromise a number of the airway management techniques available can be used. For example, an early small tonsillar carcinoma could be anaesthetized with an intravenous general anaesthetic technique. Larger tumours in the oral cavity may cause complete or partial obstruction following the induction of anaesthesia and awake fibreoptic techniques may be more suitable. Tumours involving the hypopharynx, vallecula and pyriform sinuses cause similar problems to laryngeal tumours and are discussed later.

Laryngeal tumours with no airway compromise

Early laryngeal tumours (T1 and most T2) arising from the supraglottic, glottic or subglottic regions of the larynx rarely produce airway compromise. Most of these tumours can be managed by intravenous induction of general anaesthesia and placement of a cuffed tracheal tube or laser tube. Alternatively, a supraglottic or subglottic jet ventilation technique can be employed for biopsy and laser resection.

Laryngeal tumours with airway compromise

For advanced laryngeal tumours (T4 and many T3 lesions) with significant airway obstruction and stridor at rest the options available are limited. Intravenous induction of general anaesthesia may precipitate total airway occlusion. Awake fibreoptic techniques are suitable for significant oral cavity and oropharyngeal pathology because they pass around the tumour. They are unsuitable for advanced laryngeal tumours because the fibrescope is required to pass through the tumour and leads to critical airway occlusion. Good topical anaesthesia is difficult to achieve and technically fibreoptic intubation around a vascular friable necrotic tumour is difficult. The options remaining are an inhalational induction, tracheostomy under local anaesthesia and transtracheal catheter placement under local anaesthesia.

Inhalational induction for advanced laryngeal tumours with airway obstruction is difficult and challenging. At least two anaesthetists are required and the ENT surgeon must be scrubbed and ready in theatre. Induction should take place on the operating table and is usually undertaken with sevoflurane in 100% oxygen. An oral or more usually a nasopharyngeal airway may help maintain airway patency. Induction is often slow with apnoeic periods and episodes of obstruction. Controversy exists as to the suitability of 'taking over' the patient's own spontaneous ventilation with bag, mask ventilation. The advantage of retaining spontaneous ventilation throughout is the inherent advantage of this technique. However, taking over ventilation allows a suitable depth of anaesthesia for laryngoscopy to be achieved quicker. This avoids the long periods of spontaneous ventilation waiting for an adequate depth of anaesthesia in which the patient may become unstable. The administration of muscle relaxants following confirmation of bag and mask ventilation provides optimal intubating conditions. Positive pressure bag and mask ventilation affords a degree of positive end expiratory pressure (PEEP). Whichever inhalational technique is chosen (maintenance of spontaneous ventilation or 'take over' of bag and mask ventilation) at a suitable depth of anaesthesia laryngoscopy is undertaken. The best chance of success is at the first attempt. A bougie should be immediately to hand and no more than two or three attempts made to pass a tube. Failure to intubate requires a tracheostomy.

Transtracheal catheter under local anaesthesia

Transtracheal catheter placement (Figure 24.13) under local anaesthesia at a level below the distal margin of the tumour is a recognized technique for the difficult airway. The catheter is placed usually at the level of the second or third tracheal rings, avoiding the tumour with the risk of bleeding and seeding of tumour further down the trachea. Once catheter placement has been confirmed inhalational or intravenous induction of anaesthesia is undertaken and jet ventilation through the transtracheal catheter commenced. To reduce the incidence of barotrauma associated with transtracheal jet ventilation in a patient

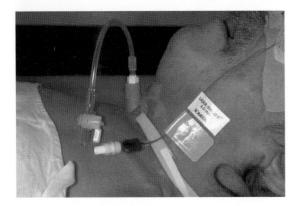

Figure 24.13 Transtracheal catheter *in situ* (sited before induction of anaesthesia).

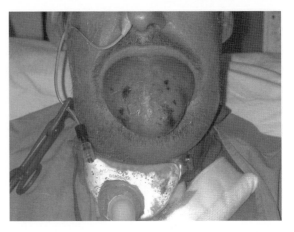

Figure 24.14 Tracheostomy under local anaesthesia (LA) required for massive tongue swelling.

with significant airway obstruction, a high-frequency jet ventilator with automatic cut-off at a preset pause pressure limit should be used and an experienced anaesthetist should remain at the head end of the patient undertaking a chin lift, jaw thrust, and use an oropharyngeal or nasopharyngeal airway as appropriate to maintain the patency of the upper airway.

Tracheostomy under local anaesthesia

The decision to perform a tracheostomy under local anaesthesia will be made in conjunction with the surgeon and will be dependent on a number of factors including the experience of the anaesthetist, the severity of the airway disease and the requirements post-resection. It can be a life-saving option in upper airway obstruction (Figure 24.14).

Tracheal obstruction

Tracheal obstruction can be caused by lesions arising within the trachea itself or by compression from surrounding structures or tumours. Two principle problems arise, first the ability to pass a tube through the obstruction and secondly difficulty siting a tracheostomy due to the location of the tumour if it is at or below the tracheostomy site. Anaesthetic management involves either intravenous or inhalational induction, fibreoptic placement of a tracheal tube with the cuff below the level of the lesion or securing the airway via rigid

bronchoscopy. Tracheobronchial stenting is an option to consider. Resection of low tracheal or carinal lesions is highly specialized work and may require cardiopulmonary bypass.

Key points

- Anaesthesia for head and neck surgery requires specialized equipment and techniques.
- Shared airway cases require careful planning between surgeon and anaesthetist.
- Use of the laser adds another hazard.
- Thorough airway evaluation includes review of CT and MRI scans.
- Review recent flexible nasendoscopy findings.
- Site of airway obstruction determines appropriate strategy.
- Take great care when employing high pressure oxygen.

Further reading

Patel A. Anaesthesia for endoscopic surgery. *Anaesth Intens Care Med* 2002; **3(6)**: 201–205.

Williams PJ, Bailey P. Comparison of the reinforced laryngeal mask airway vs tracheal intubation for adenotonsillectomy. *Br J Anaesth* 1993; **70**: 30–33.

A. Steele

Introduction

Intensive care units (ICUs) were originally developed more than 50 years ago to offer patients prolonged respiratory support. Of course, more recently there have been great advances in the support of other organs. Nevertheless, ventilation and its accompanying airway management techniques remain at the centre of intensive care practice.

Endotracheal intubation

Indications for intubation

Respiratory failure is the main indication for endotracheal intubation in the ICU. However, there are other indications, including: control of partial pressure of carbon dioxide (P_aCO_2) in head injury patients, airway protection (e.g. during endoscopy), to allow investigations (e.g. bronchoscopy, computed tomography or magnetic resonance imaging scan), for transfer to another hospital or for uncontrolled seizures. Haemodynamic instability due to septic or cardiogenic shock is also an under-recognized indication for intubation.

Decision to intubate in respiratory failure

The decision to intubate should be primarily made on clinical grounds and the figures in Table 25.1 should be used as a guideline only. As an example the patient with chronic neurological weakness managed with nocturnal bilevel positive airway pressure (BIPAP) may normally have a P_aCO_2 of 8.0 kPa and would almost certainly not require intubation. However, a young asthmatic patient who is deteriorating rapidly despite aggressive treatment may require intubation with a P_aCO_2 of only 7.0 kPa. In general terms consideration should be given to the underlying diagnosis, the possibility of improvement with intensification of treatment, the trend in the clinical picture and most importantly whether the patient is tiring.

Organizational factors such as the availability of skilled support and the time of day are also often important considerations. Respiratory function and the ability to observe changes in respiratory function are decreased at night. Most intensivists would be more inclined to intubate a deteriorating patient at night, when fewer staff are available, than they would during the day.

Ethical considerations

Timing of intubation

In some emergencies endotracheal intubation must be performed immediately to avoid increased risk to the patient's life. However, in many situations it is possible to delay intubation to allow relatives time to visit. Even a brief opportunity to talk in private can be very important for families of patients who do not survive.

Table 25.1 Criteria for mechanical ventilation

- Tidal volume <3 ml kg^{-1}
- Respiratory rate >35 min^{-1}
- Vital capacity <15 ml kg^{-1}
- FEV$_1$ < 10 ml kg^{-1}
- P$_a$O$_2$ < 8 kPa
- P$_a$CO$_2$ > 8 kPa

Withholding intubation

It is more difficult to withhold intubation than many other treatments for several reasons:

- There is usually little time in which to act.
- By the time the question of intubation arises patients are usually not competent to make a decision.
- An order to withhold intubation is clearly usually irreversible.
- Finally, it is very difficult to predict non-survival with absolute certainty.

General rules of thumb are that the patient's wishes are paramount, where possible decisions should be taken after discussion with the patient and their family, and agreement between the intensive care consultant and the referring consultant should be achieved. A decision to withhold intubation should be fully documented in the medical notes. When there is time to talk to patients, it is quite common for patients and families who initially insist on intubation to change their decision once they understand the whole intensive care treatment and weaning process.

Standard of care

The same standard of care for endotracheal intubation should apply in the ICU as in the operating theatre. Patients who have been in the ICU for more than a few days often have significant oedema of the upper airway and can be difficult to intubate. Particular points for consideration are that an appropriately skilled person (in the UK usually an anaesthetic registrar) should perform the intubation with a skilled assistant, monitoring should include capnography and the full range of difficult intubation equipment should be available. Even with very small doses of induction agents intensive care patients can become haemodynamically stable and pressor agents should be readily available.

Route of intubation

The vast majority of patients will have an orotracheal tube, followed by a tracheostomy if necessary. Nasal tubes while more comfortable than oral tubes are associated with an increased incidence of sinusitis and make tracheal toilet virtually impossible. Since the advent of percutaneous tracheostomy nasal intubation in the ICU has become a historical technique.

Tracheostomy

Indication and timing

In broad terms any patient who has failed to wean by 7–10 days will require a tracheostomy. Orotracheal intubation for >10 days has been associated with an increased incidence of laryngeal stricture. However, the precise timing of tracheostomy remains controversial and will depend on the pre-morbid condition of the patient. For example, an elderly patient with an infective exacerbation of chronic obstructive pulmonary disease would merit a tracheostomy within the first few days of admission.

Open vs. percutaneous tracheostomy

The advantages of bedside percutaneous tracheostomy over surgical tracheostomy are mainly of convenience and timing. Nevertheless, the ability to offer most patients safe, rapid tracheostomy without delay has increased the range of patients to whom long-term weaning may be offered. As a result of this percutaneous tracheostomy has in fact been one of the most important advances in intensive care practice in the last decade (Box 25.1).

The number of patients needed for a randomized controlled trial of sufficient power to compare surgical and percutaneous tracheostomy would be so high that there will always be debate over the relative advantages of the two techniques. The issue is further complicated by some surgeons who offer open tracheostomy at the bedside and others who having performed a standard surgical exposure of the anterior trachea then use a percutaneous tracheostomy set to form the stoma in the operating theatre. However, a few points can be made with reasonable certainty:

- Percutaneous tracheostomy is safe, provided the operator is properly trained and experienced.

Box 25.1 Complications of percutaneous tracheostomy

Early
- Bleeding
- Pneumothorax
- Misplaced tube (oesophageal/pre-tracheal)
- Tracheal tear
- Bacteraemia.

Intermediate
- Infection
- Erosion of innominate artery
- Tracheo-oesophageal fistula.

Long term
- Tracheal stenosis
- Hoarse voice
- Keloid scar.

- The infection rate from percutaneous tracheostomy is probably lower than from open tracheostomy.
- Percutaneous tracheostomy should not be performed in patients with unfavourable anatomy (i.e. landmarks obscured by adipose tissue or large thyroid, low lying cricoid, large veins overlying puncture site). Around 10–20% of intensive care patients are anatomically unsuitable for percutaneous tracheostomy.

Method

The various techniques for percutaneous tracheostomy are described in detail in intensive care text books. All methods rely on the placement of a guidewire below the cricoid, ideally between the first and second tracheal ring. Higher placement risks damaging the cricoid, lower placement risks exsanguination from damage to intrathoracic blood vessels. Bronchoscopy is mandatory to confirm correct placement of the guidewire and to exclude puncture of the posterior tracheal wall (and oesophageal passage of the guidewire). Ultrasound can be used to facilitate identification of the trachea and capnography applied to the penetrating needle is an alternative to bronchoscopic identification. Many practitioners find it useful to try and observe the needle actually penetrating the trachea via the endoscope, but the risk of damage to the 'scope' is much increased. Replacing the tube with a laryngeal

mask airway (LMA) or ProSeal LMA reduces this hazard.

Some operators prefer a blunt dissection technique to identify the anterior tracheal wall before passage of the needle. However this is rarely necessary and is likely to increase the risk of stomal infection over a true minimally invasive percutaneous technique.

Once the guidewire has been correctly located the trachea is dilated either by serial dilators, a tapered single dilator, a threaded screw-dilator or by fenestrated angled forceps designed to slide over the guidewire (Griggs forceps). In practice there is little to choose between the techniques. The Griggs forceps technique is the quickest but it requires considerable judgement by the operator as to the degree of force to apply. Concerns have been raised that in less-skilled hands there is a greater risk of tracheal tear with the technique. The more recently introduced tapered single dilators made by several manufacturers offer only slightly less rapid access to the trachea and are probably the commonest method in use in the UK.

Tracheostomy tubes

A size 8.0 cuffed tracheostomy tube will be suitable for most patients but larger and smaller sizes should be available. Tracheostomy tubes with internal cannulae are now obtainable at low cost and should be used as a matter of choice to prevent tracheal secretions encrusting the cannula lumen.

Changing the tracheostomy tube

Changing the tracheostomy tube in the first 5–7 days before a track has formed can be problematic and should be avoided if possible. If an early tube change is necessary, it should always be performed by someone who can rescue the airway (an anaesthetist or ENT surgeon). The patient should always be pre-oxygenated and if possible starved. A full range of intubating equipment, bougie, tracheal dilators and surgical instruments must also be available at the bedside.

Changing the tracheostomy tube after 1 week is usually straightforward. Nevertheless, care should be taken to suction oropharyngeal secretions pooled above the cuff and to perform thorough tracheal suctioning as the tube is removed. A range of smaller tubes should be immediately available.

Removal of the tracheal tube (decannulation)

General intensive care patients

The majority of patients passing through a general ICU will not have neurological or laryngeal disease. For these patients decannulation is relatively straightforward and can be performed once the following criteria have been met:

- At least 24 h breathing spontaneously via a tracheostomy mask without continuous positive airway pressure (CPAP) or other assisted ventilation.
- Low production of tracheal secretions and able to clear secretions from oropharynx.
- Able to swallow without obvious aspiration – nurse or physiotherapy supervised 'blue dye test'.

If the above conditions have been met it is safe to decannulate, and speech and language therapy referral can be avoided.

Neurological or laryngeal disease

For patients with neurological or laryngeal disease, or who have failed the above criteria the decision to decannulate is more complicated; and it will require specialist speech and language therapy, and perhaps otolaryngological advice. Although the same criteria apply, assessment and monitoring of improvement will be more difficult. Patients with chronic dysfunction may never meet the criteria and a decision will have to be made about a long-term tracheal cannula.

For patients where some recovery can be expected it will often be useful to 'down-size' the tracheostomy tube by placing a series of smaller, fenestrated tubes. This offers access for continued tracheal toilet and allows the patient to breathe and speak for periods with the tracheostomy tube 'capped off', while further assessment of swallowing occurs. The passage of air through the anatomical airway also helps recovery of the oropharyngeal and laryngeal reflexes.

Long-term respiratory support

General ICU are likely to see an increasing number of patients being weaned to nocturnal BIPAP ventilation. Once recovery from the acute illness has occurred in these patients, a useful strategy can be to move the patient gradually from 24-h pressure support ventilation (often with a deflated cuff) to pressure support ventilation at night with spontaneous ventilation during the day. Before removal of the tracheostomy tube nocturnal nasal/facial BIPAP can be started while tight tape is placed over the tube and tracheal stoma to prevent gas leakage. Although simple in principle such techniques are often complicated in practice and require highly skilled and experienced staff in all the disciplines involved. Ideally all patients requiring long-term respiratory support should therefore be transferred to a specialist long-term ventilation centre as soon as they enter the weaning phase of their illness.

Non-invasive ventilation

There has been a recent expansion in the use of non-invasive ventilation (NIV) in acutely ill patients. This has been driven both by the availability of cheap portable ventilators, improvements in mask design and the publication of a number of trials demonstrating improved outcome in selected groups of patients. Current indications for NIV are chronic obstructive pulmonary disease with respiratory acidosis, type II respiratory failure secondary to chest wall deformity or neuromuscular disease, cardiogenic pulmonary oedema and as an aid to ventilatory weaning in selected patients (Box 25.2).

Where NIV is offered but invasive ventilation is considered inappropriate then many of these contraindications will not apply.

Patient–ventilator interface

The success of NIV is dependent on the interface between the patient and the ventilator. The design of the ventilator is an important non-adjustable part of the interface but equally important is the choice of mask and headgear. The correct selection and

Box 25.2 Contraindications to NIV

- Surgery to face, airway or oesophagus
- Vomiting or profuse oral secretions
- Inability to protect airway
- Decreased conscious level
- Severe confusion
- Severe asthma
- Undrained pneumothorax.

fitting of the mask can make an enormous difference to patient compliance, and physiotherapists or nurses involved in delivering NIV must be properly trained. Even with best practice, however about 25% of patients will be unable to tolerate NIV. A poorly fitting face mask will result in the ventilator failing to detect inspiration. Subsequent attempts to tighten the mask strapping to improve mask-fit can lead to necrosis of the nasal bridge within a few days.

Recent improvements in mask design include sophisticated masks which employ cushioned gel and comfort flaps to limit air leakage. Individually moulded masks employing heat sensitive plastic and large masks which enclose the whole face are also now available. These technological advances are likely to lead to increased compliance with NIV.

Practical considerations in initiating NIV

Having identified a suitable patient, care should be taken to ensure that there are no contraindications to NIV. The patient should be able to maintain their airway, there should be minimal oral secretions and no history of recent facial or upper gastrointestinal surgery. In the acute situation a full face mask of the appropriate size is selected and time should be taken to hold the mask in place to familiarize the patient with the technique. Ventilatory support should be increased gradually from an initial setting of 5 cmH$_2$O expiratory peak airway pressure (EPAP) and 12 cmH$_2$O inspiratory PAP (IPAP) to 20 cmH$_2$O IPAP.

It is usually possible to tell within a few hours whether NIV will be successful. As the patient gradually improves, consideration can be given to converting to a nasal mask and gradually reducing periods and degree of ventilatory support over the following days. If the technique fails then the patient should be referred for invasive ventilation or a limitation of care order should be made after appropriate discussion with the patient and their family.

Bronchoscopy

Management of the airway for diagnostic bronchoscopy

Immunocompromised patients with pneumonia are occasionally referred to intensive care for monitoring during diagnostic bronchoscopy. Although bronchoscopy can be performed through a port in a face mask, usually it will be necessary to intubate such patients. Careful consideration should therefore be given to the likely utility of the information from bronchoalveolar lavage (BAL).

It is vital that during the procedure an anaesthetist manages the airway and ventilation. The only particular point of detail is that positive end expiratory pressure (PEEP) should be maintained for as long as possible. This is best achieved by using an angle piece with a rubber seal designed to pass a bronchoscope. (The alternative of simply disconnecting the catheter mount from the endotracheal tube will result in longer periods without PEEP.) The bronchoscopist must be prepared to interrupt the procedure immediately if there is any sign of destabilization. Although bronchoscopy usually results in a temporary deterioration in these patients, many will improve after a few hours of ventilation. The timing of extubation is crucial as only very few immunocompromised patients who receive ventilation for >24 h survive.

Diagnostic bronchoscopy in managing the airway

The two roles for bronchoscopy in airway management in the ICU are for percutaneous tracheostomy (described above) and for management of lobar collapse.

Collapse of a lung or lobe is a common occurrence in intensive care patients. The cause is nearly always retained secretions forming a mucous plug and it is rare for a new endobronchial lesion to present in intensive care. Bronchoscopy can be extremely effective in re-expanding collapsed areas of lung, however the effect may only be temporary even after extensive removal of secretions. In most patients bronchoscopy can in fact be reserved as second line intervention, to be used only if physiotherapy, unguided tracheal lavage and high PEEP (up to $20\,cmH_2O$) with paralysis have failed. Exceptions to this rule would be patients with critically low oxygenation despite the non-invasive measures described above or for whom BAL is, in any case, indicated for microbiological diagnosis.

Key points

- Full monitoring and the presence of appropriately experience staff are as important in the ICU as in the operating theatre when managing the airway.
- Percutaneous tracheostomy is safe provided the operator is trained and patients are selected carefully.
- Tracheostomy change in the first 5–7 days should be avoided where possible.
- Tracheostomy tubes should have an internal cannula.
- Patients without long-term neurological impairment can usually be decannulated quickly after 24 h of breathing without CPAP.
- Choice of mask and mask size are crucial to the success of NIV.

Further reading

Anon JM, Escuela MP, Gomez V et al. Percutaneous tracheostomy: Ciaglia Blue Rhino versus Griggs' Guide Wire Dilating Forceps. A prospective randomized trial. *Acta Anaesthesiol Scand* 2004; **48**: 451–456.

Craven RM, Laver SR, Cook TM, Nolan JP. Use of the Pro-Seal LMA facilitates percutaneous dilatational tracheostomy. *Can J Anaesth* 2003; **50**: 718–720.

Gwilyn S, Cooney A. Acute fatal haemorrhage during percutaneous dilatational tracheostomy. *Br J Anaesth* 2004; **92**: 298.

Mallick A, Venkatanath D, Elliot SC et al. A prospective randomised controlled trial of capnography vs. bronchoscopy for Blue Rhino percutaneous tracheostomy. *Anaesthesia* 2003; **58**: 864–868.

S.M. Yentis

Introduction

Most anaesthetists are worried about the airway in obstetrics. This worry goes back over many years to the high incidence of difficult and failed intubation/ventilation that regularly used to feature in the Reports on Confidential Enquiries into Maternal Deaths until 15–20 years ago. Partly through better training/facilities and partly through greater use of regional anaesthesia in obstetrics, the incidence of such problems in recent reports is low. However, the possibility of unexpected difficulty remains (see below) and there is concern that recent changes in anaesthetic training in the UK have led to more limited exposure of trainees to clinical anaesthesia in general, and to general anaesthesia for Caesarean section in particular, resulting in an increase in airway problems.

The airway and pregnancy

There are several reasons why problems with the airway may be more common and serious in pregnant women than in other patients. First, technical aspects of airway management are more difficult; second, management is often particularly stressful because of the urgency of the case, increasing the importance of human factors and third, the consequences of difficulty are more serious (Table 26.1).

Prediction of difficulty with the airway is notoriously inaccurate and is covered in detail in Chapter 15. Although there are many studies of prediction of difficulty, most have excluded pregnant women. The factors that might assist prediction of difficulty are thought, in general, to be the same as for non-pregnant patients.

Non-anaesthetic airway problems

Airway problems may occur as a result of pregnancy and labour alone, albeit rarely. Pre-eclampsia is common and results in oedema which may be marked, although airway obstruction in the absence of instrumentation would be rare. Airway obstruction associated with hypocalcaemia and tetany resulting from hyperventilation induced by labour pain has been described, as has surgical emphysema arising from excessive straining or pushing.

Regional anaesthesia

One advantage of regional anaesthesia, if not the main one, is the avoidance in most cases of the need for airway support. However, although regional anaesthesia has a low *incidence* of high regional blocks, the large proportion of Caesarean sections that are now done under regional anaesthesia means that the *number* of high regional blocks one would expect to see in routine practice is approximately equal to the number of failed intubations (see below). High blocks may develop insidiously and it is, therefore, important to observe the patient continuously during surgery. Even with a symptomatic high block, reassurance and oxygen may be sufficient treatment, but there should be a low threshold for tracheal intubation as outlined below.

General anaesthesia

The technique of airway management used for general anaesthesia should be a rapid sequence

Table 26.1 Technical and human factors contributing to difficulty with the airway in pregnancy, and reasons why the consequences of difficulty are greater

Technical factors	Human factors	Consequences of difficulty
• Relatively young age group; presence of a full set of teeth. • Increased weight gain in pregnancy; deposition of fat and fluid around the head and neck. • Tendency for women to receive large amounts of intravenous fluid in labour, exacerbating oedema. • Risk of developing pre-eclampsia with further fluid retention/ overload. • Worsening of facial/laryngeal oedema during labour and pushing. • Hindrance of insertion of the laryngoscope blade into the mouth caused by enlarged breasts and the assistant's hand applying cricoid pressure. • Distortion of laryngeal anatomy caused by cricoid pressure. • Nasal venous dilatation, leading to bleeding upon instrumentation.	• Inexperience of anaesthetist and assistant, related to low exposure to general anaesthesia for Caesarean section. • Haste prompted by urgency of the case. • Knowledge that two patients are at risk. • Unfamiliarity with surroundings if staff are covering labour ward from another area. • Anxiety/panic of the patient, her partner and other staff.	• Rapid hypoxaemia caused by reduced maternal functional residual capacity and increased oxygen consumption. • Increased risk of regurgitation of gastric contents and their aspiration.

induction (see Chapter 20), modified in the presence of pre-eclampsia to reduce the hypertensive response to intubation. Particular attention should be directed towards reducing the likelihood of difficulty, and reducing the severity of the consequences if difficulty occurs (Table 26.2).

Difficult and failed intubation

The incidence of these is uncertain since definitions vary (Chapter 15). The incidence of failed intubation in obstetrics is said to be approximately 1 : 300 to 1 : 800; there is general agreement however that the incidence is higher than in the non-pregnant population, for the reasons given in Table 26.1. Another contributing factor to a high reported incidence, especially recently, is that trainees are now taught to declare failure earlier rather than persist with attempts to intubate. The incidence of failed *ventilation* (by mask or other device) is unknown.

The value of a 'drill' in the management of difficult/failed intubation has long been recognized and a modern, simplified version is offered in Figure 26.1. Along with earlier declaration of 'failed intubation', noted above, is the modern emphasis on giving only a single dose of suxamethonium and performing a single laryngoscopy, rather than repeated doses/attempts that may lead to trauma and hypoxaemia (an exception might be when the vocal cords are seen fleetingly and the anaesthetist is confident that intubation is achievable at the second attempt). Although the ProSeal laryngeal mask airway has been suggested as being useful because of the ability to vent regurgitated material, most experience with salvage of potential disasters has been with the standard laryngeal mask airway. Similarly, though the intubating laryngeal mask airway may allow successful intubation, there is no evidence that it is more effective at saving life than the standard device in this situation.

Table 26.2 Approach to airway management in the obstetric patient

	Comments
Reduce likelihood of difficulty	
Prediction before anaesthesia	Difficult.
Avoiding need for general anaesthesia	Better communication; use of regional anaesthesia.
Availability of and familiarity with a range of airways, intubation aids and larygoscopes	Implications for resources and training. Smaller tracheal tubes than in non-pregnant patients (e.g. 6.0–7.0 mm) have been suggested as being easier to place and reducing trauma.
Proper positioning of patient's head/neck	May be hindered by lateral tilt used to avoid aortocaval compression. Obese patients need pillows etc placed under the head, neck and upper shoulders.
Properly applied cricoid pressure	Can be assessed and practised immediately before induction using weighing scales.
Adequate dose of induction agent and suxamethonium	To reduce awareness and improve intubating conditions respectively. Use of non-depolarizing neuromuscular blocking drugs (e.g. rocuronium) instead of suxamethonium has been suggested, since good intubating conditions are maintained for longer, but this is not generally accepted routine practice.
Well-rehearsed 'drill'	To prevent repeated attempts and airway trauma that will hinder management of the airway even further.
Reduce severity of consequences	
Use of antacids, histamine-2 antagonists and prokinetics	To reduce acidity and volume of gastric contents.
Pre-oxygenation	To prolong the period of apnoea before hypoxaemia ensues. Either 2–3 min of normal breathing or 4–5 vital capacity breaths are considered adequate. Requires a tightly fitting face piece and high fresh gas flow.
Well-rehearsed 'drill'	To maintain oxygenation.

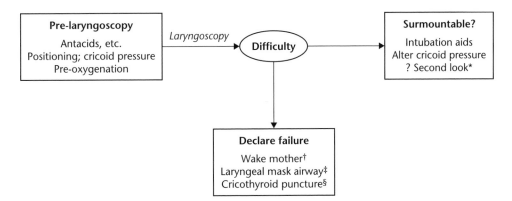

Figure 26.1 Simplified 'drill' suitable for difficult/failed intubation in obstetrics. *Standard teaching is that a second look is discouraged unless in exceptional circumstances. †Standard teaching is that the mother should always be woken unless *her* life is in immediate danger (e.g. haemorrhage), unless the foetus' life is at risk and the *anaesthetist has sufficient expertise.* ‡Some authorities advocate attempted ventilation *via* face piece/oral or nasal airway before inserting the laryngeal mask airway. Insertion of the latter may be facilitated by temporary release of cricoid pressure. §Some authorities advocate other devices (e.g. Combitube) before cricothyroid puncture.

The question of whether to proceed with an urgent case of foetal compromise without tracheal intubation (e.g. with a face mask or laryngeal mask airway), or to risk death of the foetus and allow the mother to wake, is a difficult one. In general, the primary duty of the anaesthetist to the mother should always be stressed – especially to trainees – and general anaesthesia continued only in exceptional circumstances and by an anaesthetist with adequate expertise of managing difficult cases; usually this would be an experienced consultant.

Once the mother is awake, she can be managed as for the known difficult case (below).

Care must also be taken with tracheal extubation, especially if there is a risk of laryngeal oedema, perhaps exacerbated by intubation, for example in pre-eclampsia. Deflating the cuff to ensure a gas leak around the tracheal tube when the end is obstructed can be used for reassurance before the tube is removed. The risk of aspiration is ever-present and gastric emptying with a stomach tube should be considered in emergency cases. Needless to say, observation and monitoring of the patient should continue post-operatively.

Management of the known difficult case

There has been debate over whether a patient presenting for surgery with known airway difficulty should be managed with regional anaesthesia, thereby avoiding the need for intubation, or with awake fibreoptic intubation, thereby avoiding the possibility that control of the airway might be needed in an emergency. Advocates of the former point out the apparent absurdity of meeting a difficult problem head-on when it can be simply avoided, whereas those of the latter highlight the small but serious risk of high regional block. Awake intubation itself is along standard lines, bearing in mind the likelihood that the mother may be terrified and require careful sedation; the increased nasal congestion that occurs in pregnancy; possible difficulty with transtracheal injection due to oedema; the risk of aspiration once the protective reflexes have been obtunded with local anaesthetic and the potentially hazardous systemic effects of vasoconstrictors in pre-eclampsia. If the mother has just been woken after failed intubation under general anaesthesia, she may be unable to co-operate fully.

Key points

- Airway management is more difficult and stressful in obstetrics and the consequences of difficulty are more serious, than in many other areas.
- Most problems involve general anaesthesia although airway management may be required in regional anaesthesia.
- It is important to practise a drill for difficult and failed intubation regularly.
- Problems may occur after tracheal extubation.

Further reading

Kuczkowski KM, Reisner LS, Benumof JL. Airway problems and new solutions for the obstetric patient. *J Clin Anesth* 2002; **15**: 552–563.

INDEX

Note: page numbers in *Italics* denote tables and displayed information.